Attitudes to Cancer

Attitudes to Cancer

THOMAS J. DEELEY

LONDON
SPCK

First published 1979
SPCK
Holy Trinity Church
Marylebone Road
London NW1 4DU

Printed and bound in Great Britain at
The Camelot Press Ltd, Southampton
ISBN 0 281 03663 2

Contents

Preface

The very word *cancer* provokes a fear and dread in our minds, a reaction which is not apparent with so many other diseases that we come into contact with. In this book I have attempted to detail the reasons for our current attitudes to cancer and to suggest possible ways in which these may be changed and a more rational approach made. Attitudes will be influenced by the involvement of the person concerned, and I have therefore detailed those of the doctor, the patient, the relatives, and the general public. We conclude that many of our current attitudes develop from a lack of or incomplete knowledge of the disease – a state of ignorance.

Cancer is a modern scourge which takes a heavy toll on the community and is a considerable challenge to modern medicine. Already we are making progress and many patients are cured, many have relief of troublesome symptoms, an early diagnosis brings hope of better prognosis, and our knowledge of the causes indicates that some cancers can be prevented. The fight will be more effective if we can change the existing attitudes and face up to the many problems that the disease presents.

Thomas J. Deeley
Spring 1978

Percentage of people dying from cancer for each five-year age group

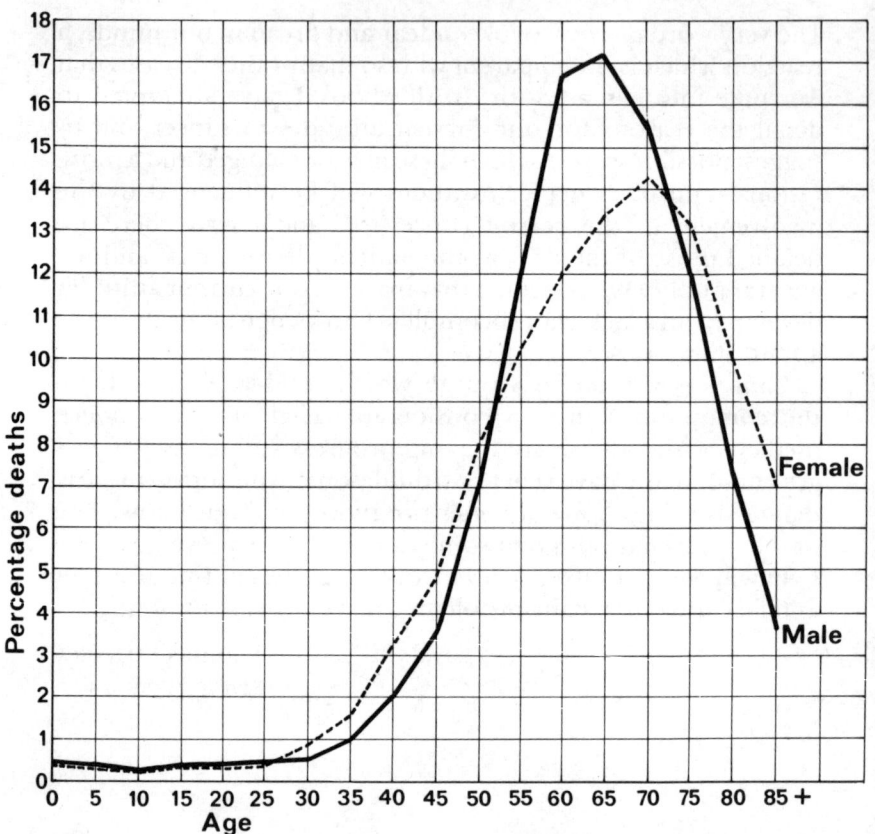

Prologue

It is not unusual to make an apology to the reader before he dips into a book. My excuse for writing this work is no more than that for many years I have cared for patients attending hospital for treatment of their cancer, full of hope that something could be done yet afraid to hear the dreaded word. Alas, too often when they came it was too late for anything more than palliation, a delay caused by the existing attitudes to the disease. We may well ask why this disease holds such a unique position in people's minds and is not treated as any other disease. To be sure, sympathy is abundant for the sufferer but it is a resigned pity analogous to that expressed for the condemned. What we need is more than pity; a rational approach to change the existing attitudes can only be based on factual scientific knowledge.

Cancer is a disease which demands a positive concerted approach. Considerable work is being done including exhaustive epidemiological studies, new diagnostic tests, greatly improved surgical, radiotherapeutic and chemotherapeutic techniques, an entirely new approach when the battle is lost, and so on. Advances are being made on a wide front and much of the work is known only to a few. Some medical practitioners, many ancillary medical staff, and the vast majority of the lay public frequently are not aware of these advances and of what can be, and is, achieved. Before we can proceed further to control cancer we must get people to accept that this is a disease which can be cured in a proportion of patients. Cancer *can* be cured, *can* be controlled, *can* be palliated, *can* be diagnosed at an early stage, and even in some cases *can* be prevented. If we can convince the public of these facts we shall bring the patient to earlier definitive care, may even detect the disease before symptoms develop, and may also institute methods of cancer prevention. I have attempted, therefore, to bring out into the light those attitudes which attend the subject of cancer, a subject that has lain hidden for too long in the shadows of mystery, magic, and ignorance. This attempt may well fail; if that is so I hope that it will at least stimulate others better qualified.

Modern attitudes to cancer have indeed developed as a garden which has been either cultivated or neglected by man through the ages. For many years the garden has been unattended and false ideas and concepts have grown like weeds and choked the facts and realities. What remains is a confused state composed of fear, disbelief, and fantasy – the present-day attitude to cancer – and these are now completely wrong. This attitude must be changed, weeds are to be removed and correct attitudes cultivated – hence my attempt.

1
Cancer

Galen (c. 130–200) was probably the first to liken a malignant tumour to a crab: 'the veins which extend from the tumour represent with it a figure much like that of a crab'; these so-called veins are strands of growth extending from the body of the tumour into the surrounding normal tissues. We use the Latin term 'cancer', or its older spelling 'canker', to describe anything which erodes, sloughs, rots, corrupts, and so on. We find it applied to a disease of trees in which the bark rots away, to a fetid affection of horses' feet, to an ulcerating lesion in the throat of fowl, to a fly which eats away fruit, and to a worm that attacks plants; in syphilis we use the word 'chancre' – again from the same source. It can be applied in a less precise way to human behaviour as in 'their word will eat as doth a canker' (2 Tim. 2.17). The word thus implies destruction, eating away, a spreading of evil or corruption.

Four aspects of the disease will be examined: the historical details, the disease process, the magnitude of the problem, and the relatively new study — oncology.

Historical Details

It has been claimed that dinosaurs suffered from cancer but the fossilized remains reveal no more than outgrowths of bone or calcified ligamentous attachments with no evidence of bone destruction. From the Edwin Smith and Ebers papyri we know that the Ancient Egyptians were familiar with the disease but there is no suggestion that it is anything more than just another disease; certainly we get no impression of fear or of a scourge.

The Greek doctor Democedes of Croton is credited with curing Atossa, the wife of Darius I (522–485 BC), who had a cancer of the breast. Here we get a first insight into a patient's reaction – she had concealed the growth for some time.

For many centuries we find little reference to the disease; epidemics, pandemics, poverty, famine, and battles all took their toll and it must be remembered that the expectation of life was short, few living to old age when malignant disease is common. The eighteenth century brought the first clue to the cause of cancer with the description of cancer of the scrotum in chimney-sweeps. We are reminded of the seriousness of the disease at this time in the first dictionary of the English language (1755) where Samuel Johnson defines it as 'a virulent swelling, or sore, not to be cured'.

The early part of the nineteenth century saw a distinct step forward with the formation of the London Society for Investigating the Nature and Cause of Cancer; by now it was a disease to be reckoned with and to deserve more study. Their inquiry, published four years later (1806) in the *Edinburgh Medical and Surgical Journal*, posed thirteen questions about the natural history of cancer.

Query 1st: What are the diagnostic signs of cancer?

Query 2nd: Does any alteration in the structure of a part take place, preceding that more obvious change which is called cancer; and if there be an alteration, what is its nature?

Query 3rd: Is cancer always an original and primary disease; or may other diseases degenerate into cancer?

Query 4th: Are there any proofs of cancer being an hereditary disease?

Query 5th: Are there any proofs of cancer being a contagious disease?

Query 6th: Is there any well marked relation between cancer and other diseases? If there be, what are those diseases to which it bears the nearest resemblance in its origin, progress, and termination?

Query 7th: May cancer be regarded at any period, or under any circumstances, merely as a local disease? Or does the existence of cancer in one part afford a presumption that there is a tendency in a similar morbid alteration in other parts of the animal system?

Query 8th: Has climate or local situation any influence in rendering the human constitution more or less liable to cancer under any form, or in any part?

Query 9th: Is there any particular temperament of body
liable to be affected with cancer more than others? If there
be, what is the nature of that temperament?

Query 10th: Are brute creatures subject to any disease
resembling cancer in the human body?

Query 11th: Is there any period of life absolutely exempt
from the attack of this disease?

Query 12th: Are the lymphatic glands ever affected
primarily in this disease?

Query 13th: Is cancer, under any circumstances,
susceptible of a natural cure?

Later the same Society stressed the different incidence of the
disease in the two sexes.

Should it be proved that women are more subject to cancer
than men, we may then inquire whether married women are
more liable to have the uterus or breasts affected; those who
have suckled, or those who did not; and the same
observations may be made of the single.

There seems no doubt that, at this time, females were
considered to have a greater incidence of the disease. John Keats
(1795–1821), in a letter dated 10 June 1818 addressed to
Benjamin Bailey, said:

Were it in my choice I would reject a petrarchal coronation –
on account of my dying day, and because women have
cancers.

The Penny Encyclopaedia of the Society for the Diffusion of Useful
Knowledge, published in 1836, has one and a half pages to cover
cancer; some quotations give us a contemporary picture:

A disease of malignant character, the real nature of which
after all the observation and research of the surgeon, still
remains wholly unknown.

It is much more frequent in the female than in the male. Its
more common seat in the female is the breast and in the male
the lips.

Of near 60 cancers, says Dr Alexander Monro, who wrote
about a century ago, which I have been present at the

extirpation of, only four patients remained free of the disease at the end of two years; three of these lucky people had occult cancer in the breast and the fourth had an ulcerated cancer of the lip.

and then:

How different the results of modern surgery!

and later:

These statements (the results of modern surgery) place in a strong light the paramount importance of attending to the very first indications of this dreadful distemper and the folly of concealing as is too often the case, especially on the part of the female, from a feeling of false delicacy, the existence of a malady which if neglected will be sure to terminate in death, attended with agonising suffering; but which if properly treated in the commencement, may be easily removed.

Thus, cancer was 'a disease to be feared', caused 'agonised suffering', and was often concealed. It is possible that many of our present-day attitudes to this disease date from beliefs founded at this time.

We come now to the the time of William Marsden (1796–1867), with his far-sighted view of a medical specialty for cancer and the need for a dedicated cancer hospital. 'Now gentlemen, I want to found a hospital for the treatment of cancer, and for the study of the disease, for at the present time we know absolutely nothing about it,' he said at the first meeting to discuss the new hospital, held on 10 February 1851. The establishment of such a hospital was fraught with problems; many people – including Queen Victoria – could not see the need for such an institution. 'Her Majesty must decline contributing to a hospital for the exclusive treatment of one disorder, the sufferers under which malady are not excluded from general hospitals,' but she relented some years later and made a generous contribution. Cancer had become a major problem.

The dawn of the twentieth century brought alarming indications of the magnitude of the disease. 'The disease is indisputably on the increase, though there is little doubt that the recognition is more frequent than it was in former days, and that greater accuracy of diagnosis now exists' (Sherman Bigg, 1907). The medical profession were aware of the need for early treatment, of the factors that affected prognosis, of the need to remove not only the tumour but the associated node areas, and they hoped for dramatic results from the promising new treatment made possible by the discovery of X-rays.

We can get some idea of the advice given to the general public from the book *Medicine for the Million. A handbook containing all the information required for ordinary purposes*, written by a 'Family Physician' and published by the *News of the World* newspaper in 1906. 'The object of this book is not to displace the family doctor but to furnish the reader with general information regarding medical subjects'; on 'Cancer' this includes: 'As to the *real immediate* causes of cancer we know almost nothing. If there is cancer in your family, you should guard against neglecting bruises, blows, sores, or inflammation of every kind; and you should, *to be quite on the safe side*, drink no alcohol and smoke no tobacco', and: 'We may lay it down, now in 1906, that nothing but early removal with the knife will give most cancer patients any chance of prolonging their lives'; but later on we see new hope: 'The X-ray method seems to promise us help in the future'.

M. Donaldson summed up the current feelings in 1933, in *Radiotherapy in the Diseases of Women*:

> At the present time cancer is taboo. It is not difficult to understand why there is such a universal fear of the disease. The public believe that it must end fatally and it appears to come like a bolt from the blue without any serious symptoms as a warning. The unfortunate victims go back to their homes, where their suffering is witnessed by the whole family during many weeks, if not months.

Young people of the time who got this impression from their parents have now themselves reached an age when cancer is a relatively common disease.

The Disease Process

We may firstly marvel at the mysteries of the human body; embryology reveals an awesome story. Two germ cells from two individuals are joined and divide along a directed path until a new individual is created; the possibilities of error are tremendous, yet we see few mistakes. The established organism then functions in a predetermined pattern, grows, matures, and reaches adulthood. We may marvel that such a complicated system can go on for so many years without dysfunction. We have only to consider the problems that arise from the continuous use of complicated mechanical or electrical machinery to appreciate the wonders of a living organism as complicated as man. And, remember, we understand the physiological and biochemical functions of the body only imperfectly, consider a heart that beats some thirty-two million times a year and which, should it stop even once, would bring about death: cells that die and are replaced by *controlled* growth millions of times in a lifetime, electrical impulses that pass and repass through the nervous system unfailingly: glands that secrete infinitesimal amounts of chemicals which control the whole body functions; the list is endless. When, in our relative ignorance, we consider the marvellous complexity of our bodily organization it seems a miracle that we should even live at all, more so that we should continue to function day after day with few or no faults. So much for the normal.

In some as yet unexplained way, there is a breakdown in the normal replacement programme. A cell replacing a dead one is not controlled and goes on dividing, and forms two cells, each of which again divides to give four, and then eight, sixteen and so on – a process of exponential growth. There is no longer *control* of the process. This growth is at first invisible and produces no symptoms, and remains so until it reaches a definite size that is visible, can be palpated, or presses on a neighbouring tissue. Each cell in this mass is *uncontrolled* and will continue to grow even if the cause which excited the breakdown is removed.

Causative factors are probably acting in all people and we wonder why some develop cancer and others not. Death from other causes may supervene, or perhaps some individuals have an inborn susceptibility to malignant change and others a resistance; some individuals will be exposed more to exciting causes than others; alternatively the body may react and fight the process and we have some clinical evidence that there are self-healing cancers.

Our knowledge of malignant diseases is at present elementary and superficial; often we are dealing with the unknown or that which is only partially appreciated. Our ignorance probably accounts for the attitudes which exist today.

The Magnitude of the Cancer Problem Today

It is difficult to get a true indication of the number of people who develop cancer each year; it is not a registerable disease and our only indication of its incidence is obtained from studies of mortality. About one-fifth of all deaths are due to cancer; it is the second commonest cause of death, surpassed only by cardiovascular diseases. We must remember that many of the deaths recorded as cardiovascular are, in fact, diseases of old age, such as hardening of the arteries, a failure of the heart muscle, or incompetence of the valves, in other words, the failure of the human machine and a natural way of dying.

Cancer has assumed this ominous position because of the important advances that have been made in curing or preventing so many other diseases that killed man before he could reach old age. Improvements in infant welfare have reduced the appalling number of deaths seen at the beginning of this century. New surgical techniques and better anaesthetics have made surgery safer and it is possible to carry out more extensive life-saving operations. Once fatal diseases, such as diabetes, are now controlled. Antibiotics have abated the number of deaths from infection, improved hygiene and public health measures have had a marked effect; even as I write we are aware that smallpox has been virtually wiped out – so we can go on. The result is that people can now expect to live to a greater age; we are in fact an ageing population and cancer is a disease which should be more commonly found in the elderly patient. The graph on page viii shows the number of people dying from cancer, the peak being over the age of fifty-five.

Whilst so many medical improvements have been made, there has not been a commensurate improvement in cancer treatment or prevention, and this has served to exacerbate the relative importance of the disease. Thus, cancer has assumed the position in our minds that tuberculosis once had, or diabetes before that, or pneumonia, appendicitis, yellow fever, cholera, leprosy, smallpox, or the Black Death had years ago. It is our modern-day scourge.

Oncology

In the past each doctor has approached malignant diseases in the light of the specialized branch of medicine that he pursues. Thus, the general practitioner meeting a patient whom he suspects has a malignancy will refer that patient to the specialist whom he thinks can best deal with diagnosis and treatment. Division of responsibility becomes involved within the hospital; each consultant sees the patient and his disease in a different way, as a diagnostician, a pathologist, a surgeon, a radio-therapist, and so on. Thus, each doctor develops an interest in one aspect of malignancy.

But these diseases constitute a small part of a doctor's whole spectrum of knowledge and interest; the urologist will meet only a relatively small number of patients with malignant diseases, so also the gynaecologist, the surgeon, the physician, the pathologist, and so on. Only the radiotherapist spends the majority of his time dealing with malignancy. Too frequently doctors take a rather limited view of the whole spectrum and are often unaware of the advances being made in other specialties.

Current thinking has broadened our horizons and we now seek information of all aspects of malignant diseases, adopting the term 'oncology' to describe the studies of tumours, derived from the Greek *onkos* – a mass, bulk, or tumour – and *logos* – science or study. Thus an oncologist is a person who studies tumours. This new study does not imply a new medical specialty and indeed it is ridiculous to think that any one doctor could practise in this way. Rather, oncology is a concept, a com-prehensive knowledge of all facets of tumours. Therefore, it embraces epidemiology, aetiology, diagnostic procedures, pathology, surgery, radiotherapy, chemotherapy, the specialist branches of clinical medicine such as gynaecology, urology, paediatrics, ear, nose and throat diseases, to name but a few, and also aftercare. Such a catholic approach to malignant diseases will help the individual doctor to practise better his own sphere of specialization. Oncology as a subject encourages us to look for the best method of patient management, unbiased by our own skills or facilities. One of the big problems has been to disseminate knowledge from one branch to another. Oncology covers a very wide range of knowledge not only in content but also in depth; it provides the means whereby workers in diverse fields, which may appear to be completely isolated from each other, may be brought together to work to one common end.

Now this demands a reappraisal of the doctor's role. We must admit that to some extent this has been in the past somewhat that of a demigod, who seeks information, sifts it, pronounces, and gives advice – any ensuing credit or blame being given to the doctor. Whilst the ultimate responsibility for medical care rests, and will always rest, with the doctor there is a great need for him to seek information and help in the care which he ultimately prescribes. Oncology does not reduce his responsibility in any way; rather it seeks to improve his knowledge and to suggest a way in which he may use this to improve his treatment. It is important that the doctor's attitude of mind seeks always for more information, more co-operation.

2
Attitudes

The word 'attitude' is used so frequently that it has become rather a loose term; it is applied correctly to posture or body position but may also be applied to the mind to define a state of thought or feeling. While it is essentially a personal attribute experienced by one individual only, yet similar exciting processes experienced by a community may produce a group response or community attitude.

Such attitudes are composed of two parts. We have basic human attitudes experienced in increasing order of complexity from primitive mammals, to primal human societies, through uneducated communities to sophisticated modern man. These attitudes are fundamental reactions and are composed of such basic factors as fear and anxiety. Such basic attitudes are strongest in the child who, as it grows, gains experience and knowledge which will attenuate them; later, therefore, the mature adult attitudes will have still some basic element, but this is greatly affected by ensuing environmental factors. Attitudes may be affected by the experiences of others, by what we are told or read, rather than what we participate in personally. Our personal responses can be influenced by others in this way if we allow it, but we can also resist such outside interference, developing our own response as a result. Our personal knowledge of the person supplying this information affects our acceptance of it far more than we realize. If our personal feelings are strong, based on experience, they are more unlikely to be affected by what we are told or read than if we have merely a negative attitude. Thus education must be forceful, positive, and acceptable if we are to change an existing attitude, whereas it is more likely to succeed, even if the information is incorrect, where no positive attitude exists. We see this exemplified when we compare the education of children and that of the adult. The child with his receptive mind is easier to teach than the adult – easier to mislead or to correct. Our attitudes may be further influenced by imagination which may fill gaps which have occurred in our perception. Usually our thoughts are controlled by personal criticism but, should this be missing, an association of ideas may take an uncontrolled course and lead to dreams or fancy, a world of imagination, which can be associated with a factual or real situation but may lead to illusion or hallucination. Our attitudes may be influenced by certain sentiments, aesthetic, religious, moral, and so on. We therefore build up a complex pattern of personal attitudes which are affected by personal experience, with the result that we get a progressive change from childhood to maturity influenced by foregoing events. The vast majority of humans are gregarious and so we get similar patterns of attitude in a group; there is seldom the wide variation that we find in individuals, and communal attitudes become those which are acceptable to all members of the group. Such attitudes determine the response conduct of a community, its culture or folk-lore, its government, response to illness, response to the unknown. But the community could uphold an attitude which would not survive in the 'individual': some communities adopt unusual or eccentric beliefs purely because of the support of numbers, and we may observe rather unusual responses to illness and suffering which either support an ascetic approach or deny the need for medical interference. Such attitudes could be broken down by reasoning with the individual but this is less likely to succeed in a community.

The mind, in its perception of experiences, will often form certain associations as a result of knowledge or of hearsay. Accordingly we have the belief that 'cancer', 'suffering', and 'death' are either synonymous or associated; this association of ideas can be passed on to others and becomes an 'accepted fact'. Perversely, where knowledge is deficient and where fear exists in the mind there is a readier acceptance of the fatal or adverse circumstance than there is of the propitious; this can in part be attributed to an innate desire, as exemplified in literature, pathos always appealing most to the audience.

Our attitudes to malignant disease are a complex mixture of basic ideas, hearsay, personal experience, and historical events. If we look back into history we find that there have existed many scourges of mankind which in their time have produced the same attitudes of mind as we now find with cancer. Included are plague, which decimated populations until the rat vector was discovered and stricter public health control greatly reduced the incidence; smallpox, and cholera, controlled by public health measures; tuberculosis, syphilis and less serious infections controlled by antibiotics, diabetes by insulin, and so on. Control of a scourge has drastically changed the attitude of the public. It needs, however, a drastic change to take place in the treatment, resulting in a vast majority of patients recovering, before marked changes in attitudes occur. Even then attitudes lag behind medical advances, and it may take some generations before the ideas instilled in the mind are changed. In malignant diseases we have certain problems; not all are cured, and often those who are cured do not know the true nature of the disease; inevitably the general public is aware of cancer only when a person dies and then people build up the association of ideas we have noted previously. We have a further complication that cancer is a generic name for a whole group of diseases ranging from very rapidly growing tumours to ones which may take years to develop and which may not shorten life expectation; it is to be expected that there is a tendency to accept the rapidly growing ones as being representative of the whole group.

We shall examine the current attitudes to cancer in four groups of people respectively – doctors, patients, relatives, and the general public. Inevitably what relates to the doctor will apply also to the other groups to a certain degree; therefore, we shall look closely at the doctor, indicating the full range of attitudes possible, and will then specify particular facets for the other three groups.

Current Medical Attitudes to Cancer

The doctor's attitude to disease is made up of two parts: a basic human attitude and that which has developed as a result of his particular training. It will inevitably change over the years; whilst young he may be greatly influenced by basic factors but, as he grows older and learns more, he will be influenced by his own experiences. Specialization in a particular branch of medicine produces a further influence on his approach; it may cause him to accept the view that cancer is inevitably a terminal disease, or he may be able to produce evidence to the contrary.

Attitudes are personal, each doctor reacting in a different way; but even so there is a group response which may be large and poorly-defined, or narrow because he is dedicated to the care of the cancer patient or more so of a particular malignancy. An analysis of medical attitudes will, of necessity, call for criticism of the doctor's approach; it is hoped that any offence which the individual doctor may feel will be balanced by his appreciation of the facts and the need to improve the current attitudes. We will therefore unreservedly use such terms as ignorance, fear, complacency, and so on, with the hope that, should they be applicable, the individual doctor will take steps to examine his own ideas, knowledge, and personal attitudes, and to correct them as may be necessary whenever possible. It is, of course, easy to be critical of others, to attribute to them any errors which have occurred, to blame them either directly or obliquely for the present-day attitudes which prevail towards malignant disease. But it is necessary to be critical if we are going to appraise any situation and benefit as a result.

We are all guilty, in varying degrees, of thinking that cancer is other than a natural disease which will respond to established methods of control, and few of us will find that the attitudes to be described are inapplicable to us.

We will look into the attitudes found in doctors, dealing first with somewhat basic attitudes shared with other members of the community, and then with more specific factors which are more relevant to the clinician.

BASIC ATTITUDES

The order of referring to these attitudes caused me much concern; they should progress, if possible, from basic human responses to the more refined thoughts resulting from clinical experience. I have therefore started with a basic human emotion – fear – and will proceed to cover more complex ideas rather in the manner of a thesaurus.

Fear

This is one of the primitive emotions which fall into fairly well-defined groups as described by F. Ryland in *The Story of Thought and Feeling* (1900):

1. Pleasure, joy, delight, satisfaction, content.
2. Pain, grief, sorrow, regret.
3. Fear, terror, horror, anxiety, apprehension, suspicion.
4. Anger, dislike, hatred, envy, malice, jealousy.

5. Affection, sympathy, love, benevolence, esteem, respect, veneration.
6. Pride, vanity, conceit, self-esteem, ambition.
7. Surprise, wonder, amazement, curiosity, admiration.

Notice the grading of these emotions, from basic to subtle. Fear exists as a very elementary form, but apprehension and suspicion are obviously more complex and imply a certain amount of knowledge and experience.

I have used the word fear as a generic term to cover all the associated emotions; it is, of course, rather an extreme form and perhaps overstresses the doctor's response and other terms may be more applicable, such as alarm, dread, horror, intense dislike, anxiety, concern, uneasiness, apprehension, suspicion, notion, inkling, and so on. These have been roughly arranged in decreasing order of severity of the emotion. The reader will be able to fit his own level to the emotion he feels at the thought of cancer. But, because they all describe a basic type of emotion, it will be convenient to refer to the whole range under the single term *fear*.

The very thought of malignant disease causes concern to us all. J. S. Mitchell says: 'One must recognise the difficulty that cancer is a subject about which few people, including doctors, can think without emotion' (*Cancer, If Curable Why Not Cured?* 1971). Part of this fear is inherent in our human make-up, a feeling that is expressed for any disease which is thought to have a hopeless prognosis, to cause suffering and pain, disability, disfigurement, distress, and so on. In part it is a response to the unknown, to the imagined; the medical practitioner may have a varied response, his experience of patients with disease may further accentuate his fear, but, alternatively, it may in part conceal it or even expel it.

His experience of cancer may be of personal disease and only few practitioners will have had that. Many doctors will have successfully repulsed the emotional entanglement associated with personal symptomatology which 'could be', 'must be' and 'quite definitely is' a malignant disease – until successfully diagnosed as being due to something else. Practically every medical practitioner has felt the panic, fright, funk, horror, despair, dread, apprehension, alarm, or whatever one likes to call it, which comes with the first realization of symptoms or signs suggestive of cancer. It is inevitable that he accepts the smallest possibility as being fact and a further consideration of the improbability will often only increase his fear. Small wonder then that his approach to the patient is somewhat coloured by his own interpretations and fears.

Experience may be gained from personal knowledge of relatives and friends who have had malignant disease; successful treatment and cure will produce one philosophy whilst at the other end the repeated frustration engendered by recurring hope and distress associated with unsuccessful treatment will invariably bring with it despondency, cynicism and despair – a response which may well moderate the clinician's attitude to his patient-care.

Finally we must accept the influence of the clinician's experience of his patients' response to therapy. It may be that he has been unfortunate in his experience; a series of patients who show an adverse response will lead him to conjecture the hopelessness of the condition in others. Another clinician may have an entirely opposite experience – a series of favourable responses to a treatment may lead him to accept that therapy with, perhaps, some complacency.

An attitude of fear may be instilled also from one's teacher. This is an emotion that is easily recognized in another and may be passed on in lectures, tutorials, or ward rounds, by tonal inflections, by subconscious stress or accentuation, or alternatively by taciturnity.

We can conclude that the doctor is a human being, who fears in the same way as his patient about any affliction which is thought or known to have a fatal and unpleasant outcome; this basic feeling may be influenced, however, by knowledge obtained from reading or from personal experience. Emotions need not overrule judgement, but we cannot escape the possibility that they may influence it.

Ignorance
Here again we use a generic term to describe a whole range of ideas. It is a somewhat derogatory term, especially when applied to professional people, but again it is the extreme end of the range and so is suitable to cover all degrees; thus ignorance, unawareness, incomprehension, inexperience, unacquaintance, unfamiliarity, rawness, naivety, and innocence may represent rather crudely the varying degrees of ignorance.

The doctor will be able to fit himself into this scale on almost any medical problem and few practitioners will be satisfied with their medical knowledge. Medicine is based on initial teaching onto which the doctor adds his unique experience derived from observation, careful recording, analysis and, to a certain degree, on trial and error resulting in an individual approach and a personal medical philosophy. Of necessity there will be gaps in both aspects – initial training and in what is subsequently added. The medical curriculum is forever increasing in coverage and depth and we may well criticize its development away from the apprentice system of clinical teaching to the more exact scientific approach. It is difficult to get the correct balance but at any rate we do produce doctors able to deal with people and interested to learn more.

The newly-qualified doctor may be excused from vainly imagining he 'knows all' should he be foolish enough to consider that he does. More usually he appreciates that he knows sufficient of the essentials to prevent him making mistakes; what he does not know he can discover in medical literature and he can get further advice when this is needed. Experience coming with years reveals to him how little he really knows, how medical knowledge to date has merely 'scratched the surface', and how much more there is to learn. Specialization with its knowledge in depth increases the desire to know more but the more man knows, the more he realizes his ignorance.

Specialization inevitably prevents the application of the same degree of concentration in other subjects. We thus have two alternatives; that of studying a great number of medical subjects each to a relatively superficial depth, or knowing one subject to a great depth and consequently not keeping up to date in all the others. Our medical knowledge, therefore, is incomplete and it is inevitable that much of our approach to a particular disease is affected by this; he that specializes in that disease contending a philosophy which cannot be shared in the same way by the vast majority of us who have no such knowledge. This is particularly so with cancer which we can now consider more fully, looking at aspects of training throughout the doctor's life.

THE DOCTOR IN TRAINING
The young medical student needs to know the problems of cancer, its prevalence, and the high toll it takes every year, and

some knowledge of its treatment and prognosis. There are few diseases where delay produces such catastrophic results and the doctor should be encouraged to refer all patients with suspicious signs or symptoms as early as possible. This is a subject which requires much research, especially clinical research, and the will to investigate must be instituted early on in the doctor's career; the student of today may well go on to solve our problems.

It is claimed that the curriculum of the medical schools is already greatly overloaded with topics which are essential to medical study, and there can be no doubt about this. We are continually adding on new information but perhaps the time has come for a reappraisal of some of the information which was basic and considered essential some twenty or so years ago but which may appear, now, to have little relevance to the clinical practice of medicine. Today, many more scientists are employed both in the hospital and associated laboratories, and it is possible that the medical student would, perhaps, benefit from less instruction about those practical and technical processes carried out more efficiently by scientists, so that he can concentrate more on the clinical application of such tests.

Undergraduate education has essentially an individualistic approach by each university and time spent on basic work, whilst appearing excessive in some medical schools, may be insufficient in others. Topic teaching, at present being adopted or investigated at some centres, offers opportunities for a correct balance of theoretical, laboratory, and clinical teaching, and is well adapted to the teaching of oncology.

We must request more training in certain branches of oncology. It is not the function of the medical school to attempt to teach surgical, radiotherapeutic, or chemotherapeutic techniques; these belong correctly to specialized postgraduate training. It is important, however, to teach basic facts, recognition of early symptoms, possible methods of early diagnosis, the optimum treatment regimes which may be used and – important – a realization that something can be done, with an appreciation of the possible outcome. It is essential that the medical school training does not instil a nihilistic approach which will result in pessimism.

THE SPECIALIST IN TRAINING

We are only a little concerned here with the training of the specialist who will spend the rest of his life in the study of tumours – the oncologist. He should have not only a deep knowledge of the particular aspect of oncology he is interested in, for example, epidemiology, pathology, diagnostic techniques, surgery, radiotherapy, and so on, but will also acquire a catholic view of the whole of his subject and the associated and adjacent disciplines – this really is the concept of oncology which is at present receiving much attention.

Malignant disease cuts across every branch of medicine and it becomes increasingly necessary that the specialist in any medical field is alerted to be aware of malignancy and has some knowledge of oncology.

KEEPING UP-TO-DATE

Teaching after qualification is somewhat less well-organized and may consist of little more than the occasional lecture to medical practitioners. The postgraduate centres have done much to improve this and many postgraduate organizers are well aware of the part that malignant disease plays in general practice and arrange for some aspects of oncology to be presented to the practitioner. Further information is obtained from current journals, reviews, annotations, and text books. Recent years have seen the growth of magazines and books specifically aimed at the general practitioner; such publications specifically omit the techniques of diagnosis and treatment, which are the province of the specialist, but aim to provide knowledge that has not been provided in undergraduate training.

We need, also, to continue the training of those doctors who specialize in the care of patients with malignant diseases. This is achieved by means of specialist meetings, seminars, and publications. Medical education is thus a continuing process.

Medical ignorance is not an intentional state; it most frequently is an act of omission rather than of commission. There are two obvious remedies: either to provide sufficient education in the undergraduate years to give at least a basic knowledge of malignant disease and to awaken an interest which will persist into postgraduate life, or alternatively to give adequate postgraduate education in the years immediately after qualification to cover the deficiency. The former is obviously preferable, but in any case continuing education should always be provided. Because of the enormity of the problem of malignancy, adequate instruction should be mandatory. The problem is obviously that of obtaining sufficient time, especially in the formative years.

Pessimism

Regrettably, no amount of education at whatever stage of the doctor's career can remove the profound pessimism felt by some doctors about this disease. We have used the word pessimism here to include the feeling of hopelessness, discouragement, defeatism, despair, despondency, the feeling that whatever is done for the patient cannot be successful because: 'Well! It's cancer isn't it', as if nothing more need be said. Such pessimism has a distinct association with cancer; doctors who are normally optimistic in their medical approach and will view many mortal diseases with a high degree of hope behave illogically where malignant disease is concerned and display no such sanguine expectations.

Pessimism may be of two kinds: inherent in the individual or resulting from experience and knowledge. It seems likely that certain individual attributes are inherited; certainly we find a family predisposition to behaviour and this is applicable to both optimism and pessimism. Man is generally optimistic; thoughts of pessimism, being fleeting only, are associated more with literature and the writers where it is 'frozen' in print for posterity. In practice, whilst many of us have pessimistic moods, these are overcome by fluctuations in the opposite direction and by factual developments.

We must therefore search for the cause of pessimism in the minds of some clinicians and without doubt this has been instilled by practical experience of the disease. Admittedly, this may be fortuitous or the physician may have a personality make-up which forces him to pay more attention than would another; this then accounts for individual variations in response. The result of a series of hopeless prognoses leads the clinician to expect this outcome: 'It's not worth trying to do anything because the outlook is hopeless in any case' – prejudgement arising out of experience. Again: 'I never send patients for radiotherapy until I think there is nothing more to be done', because radiotherapy cannot achieve the impossible at this late stage in the disease the result is a confirmation of the clinician's original belief about the hopelessness of the disease – but, the mistake in the logic is that the patient was sent too late. The surgeon and the radiotherapist may also be to blame; strong belief in a certain method of treatment, the occurrence of an unexpected recovery or 'a miracle' leading to excessive or uncalled for optimism tends to promote treatment of more advanced lesions, and the surgeon or radiotherapist is tempted to 'have a go' on the hopeless case. Naturally this is not good propaganda for his technique, a fatal outcome is what everyone expected and this may well be confirmed if he attempts the impossible.

The doctor who refers the patient for such treatment is not impressed and so he delays sending the next similar patient. Thus, over-optimism in the mind of the therapist may result in patients being referred not earlier but, paradoxically, later.

Once this pessimistic approach has taken root – be it no more than a feeling, a collection of anecdotal occurrences (and we must be aware of the part such single occurrences play in shaping our philosophy), or whether there is factual proof – once established it needs a great deal of persuasion to change. Logically we should be able to present the clinician with factual data to support a more optimistic approach. Statistics unfortunately are frequently viewed with suspicion by the average doctor; an attempt to prove a useful outcome of anti-cancer therapy often only achieves the opposite result when imperfectly understood and statistical details only 'confuse the issue'. Admittedly much of this results from an ignorance of statistical methods and their application. To change the thinking of the clinician we need a straightforward appraisal of fact, given simply without ambiguity – the best way of doing this is, of course, in the combined clinic where the pessimistic clinician can himself see the patient at follow-up. It is important to stress here the 'combined clinic' – therapist and referring clinician see every patient together, and each doctor benefits from the other's opinion. Unfortunately combined clinics often degenerate into simultaneous clinics, each doctor seeing patients individually in separate rooms and only consulting when there is a problem or a rather interesting or unusual case. Little is gained in these clinics apart from the convenience of having a colleague on hand who may help in the disposal or care of the patient.

A further point must be made; unfortunately the pessimist is not content even with a high proportion of cures. In his mind the disease is either cured, or treatment is unsatisfactory; it is an all or none response where degree does not matter. Whilst he does not apply this philosophy to many branches of medicine he unfortunately seems to in malignant disease. Again, he tends to remember and to take notice of the patients who are not cured and to disallow those who are. Even in cancer of the skin with its high cure rate it can be noted that many clinicians tend to remember the failures rather than the successes. We all have a tendency to remember ancedotal details rather than to take an overall view.

Resignation

Somewhat similar to but not exactly the same as pessimism is resignation, a feeling of submission, passiveness, capitulation or surrender, which, though not taking a fatalistic attitude to malignancy, accepts it and makes no attempt to institute treatment or to determine ways of improving existing results. This philosophy accepts that what is, is God's will, and that nothing we can do can alter it.

Whilst such doctors will have every sympathy for the patient and will do everything in their power to assist him, to relieve him of pain and worry and stress, they do not believe that anything useful can be done and so do not refer him or delay sending him for more active treatment. Such practitioners believe that the mental trauma of referral for mutilative surgery or radiotherapy, or the very realization that he has malignant disease, is more repulsive to the patient than his actual acceptance and subsequent fight for cure. Admittedly the concept of the cancer ward or hospital is often summed up 'all hope abandon, ye who enter here'.

It is totally illogical to accept in this way that nothing can be done, to be resigned to a fate; this is against all thoughts of human progress. A wise doctor may be resigned when death is at hand or when he makes a decision not to continue active therapeutic measures, but to pre-empt the outcome, especially when the patient is relatively fit, stems only from a lack of knowledge and experience.

Indifference

Closely allied to resignation is indifference, where the facts can be ignored because of a lack of interest or apathy. Relevant to cancer this can occur in two ways; firstly it may be that initial interest has not been encouraged, that one's colleagues and teachers have shown no interest, that experience has led us to believe that there is nothing to be done or, secondly, if it is done, the total effect on the patient is not satisfactory and he would have been better left alone. These views are an accumulation in part of the attitudes we have already discussed: fear, ignorance, pessimism, and resignation.

Another form of indifference arises out of preoccupation; this is a fault that all medical practitioners cannot fail but fall prey to at some time. Medicine has now got so broad and needs such expert knowledge that few of us have the time to read broadly and obtain a catholic view. Specialization has further added to our problems, there is so much to learn, to research into, even in the smallest branch of medicine, that little time can be spared for reading outside our main interest.

Again, we must go back to training; if there is never any stimulation to study malignant diseases in the formative years there is a small chance of ever developing it. Continuing interest must be maintained by pertinent reminders in the literature, designed not for the erudite specialist but for those who are merely interested enough to want to keep up. It is much easier to write on a specialized subject for the specialist than it is to write for 'the others' and to make it interesting enough for them to read.

Still a further type of indifference is that which suggests that soon a pill will be discovered which will cure cancer – a panacea to be obtained from any chemist: 'It won't be long now so why waste time trying to do anything until it is on the market.' Ignorance and indifference show certain similarities.

Lack of Interest

There can be little doubt that certain medical specialties appear more glamorous than others, especially so to the student in training; inevitably he will develop an interest in those parts of the medical curriculum which stimulate his initial interest. In addition he will show more interest in those aspects of medicine which are encouraged, sponsored or perhaps dramatized by certain members of his medical school. Thus, the work of academic departments appears more worthwhile than that of the more mundane service units. The study of cancer and some other diseases may appear dull, boring, or monotonous, producing little or no reward as judged by the number of cures or improvements in the patient's general condition. As far as many members of the general public are concerned the subnormal, the mental defective, the old and the cancer patient are best forgotten; they accept that such conditions occur and: 'Thank goodness there are places for such people should they be unfortunate enough.' Not surprising, then, that these subjects do not achieve the same academic status as do some other medical specialties and that others view the work of these specialties as anything anyone can do, lacking in specialized skill, and therefore a somewhat inferior branch of medicine. Here, I must admit that I am thinking as a radiotherapist and detailing the attitudes taken by some medical colleagues when discussing my own specialty. It is unfortunate that many people (lay and medical) think that there is little more in radiotherapy than palliation. It is surprising that intelligent people, who should know better because they are in positions of authority, dismiss any cures or survivals as being radiotherapy propaganda produced to encourage the workers in the department to carry on their work – surprising? Yes! but it is true.

Allied with this uninterested approach is the feeling that cancer is not a suitable subject for discussion – in modern jargon 'non-U'. Admittedly many are interested in cancer research provided that this remains in the laboratory and is limited to animals and chemicals in test-tubes but – please! – not patients. Some years ago two other diseases also enjoyed this taboo, tuberculosis and venereal diseases; but, changes have occurred, the fear and mystique have been removed from tuberculosis; sex and venereal diseases are now common talk, nay! requisite talk for our modern enlightened permissive society, with no longer the shame or embarrassment which called for drawing aside and whispers. But, *cancer*, we never mention that if we can avoid it and if we do there is an added aura of mystery.

I do realize that I may have overdramatized, but there is more than an element of truth in it and many of us have felt this way at some time or other.

A Depressing Subject

There is a popular belief that cancer is a depressing subject and that this is more than workers can bear and surely they will eventually break down with the very burden of depression. Who would want to deal with such a morbid subject? But, what of morbid anatomy, of forensic medicine, or undertaking, of embalming? This is different, of course, because here all life has gone. We are dealing with a corpse which has no suffering, no distress. Not so with cancer where the clinician is always present at a time when all hope is gone or almost gone, when suffering is at its worst, when the frail body has reached its limits of endurance – certainly we have a difference, the difference between a corpse and a tragedy. Admittedly there are times of depression in the life of anyone intimately concerned with the care of the cancer patient; but, this is true of most branches of medicine where we are dealing with disease, suffering, and pain. The feeling of depression is worse when dealing with the young patient, not so much perhaps with the infant who has not yet blossomed out and retains his innocence of life but with the child or teenager who is on the brink of discovering life, vital, curious, blossoming forth ready to assume manhood. Cancer in these adolescents leaves a bitter taste and at this time it is usual for those involved to feel depressed, to regret, but invariably this is followed by the desire to fight, to conquer. Cancer in old age is familiar, a frequent occurrence; the race has been run and now the end approaches, no depression, no regrets, only a desire to ease, to comfort, and to make the passing as comfortable and dignified as possible.

The stimulus to carry on the fight is accentuated when we see a patient who is cured and returns to his normal life and responsibility, or when a virulent growth is controlled: more so when the unexpected occurs, the apparently hopeless patient given palliation treatment who responds almost miraculously. But, miracles are for some only, and not all of us believe in them. Logically it would appear to be a mere case of probabilities, of mathematical and statistical analysis; however small the chance of something happening, if there are sufficient numbers that chance will eventually occur. But if we relied on miracles alone there would be little of interest in cancer therapy and we might truly say that it was depressing. The study of cancer is far from depressing, there is so much to investigate, so much to improve, so many rewards in seeing a victory achieved.

Complacency

There is yet another aspect, that of complacency. This in part stems from a feeling of satisfaction that because the disease is not curable the physician is content that he is doing the best possible; and, as a result, he may assume sufficient indifference to ignore the literature and not keep up with new developments. In part it is associated with smugness: 'I have considered all the possibilities and have decided that my way is best or at least no worse than any other, I have it under control', or further: 'This is how I treat; I did this exactly the same last year and the year before and so on right to the time when I first encountered the disease.' We are all well aware of this self-satisfied approach to medicine; in the days of increasing medical knowledge it is false to feel able to cope with even one disease. The opposing view, a dissatisfaction with the existing results of treatment, is closely allied to *research* and *development*, the means by which we will eventually control the disease. Suffice it here to say that as far as malignant disease is concerned there is, at the present state of our knowledge, absolutely no place for even a trace of complacency.

Conclusion

The factors responsible for the present attitudes to malignant disease have such a close relationship to each other that it becomes impossible to distinguish them separately; thus, indifference is often associated with ignorance, as is pessimism. Fear at first appears to be unique but here again ignorance may further affect it or attenuate it to a large degree. The presence of one factor frequently opens up the possibility of another exerting an influence; it then becomes difficult to determine which came first and which exerts the most influence. These combinations and permutations result in a complex individual response; although the same factors may be present in two doctors the results and responses to cancer may be widely different. Of all the factors influencing our attitudes to malignant disease the most important is assuredly ignorance – it is something about which we should have no pride but it can be remedied, provided, of course, that suitable facilities are available. Once committed to the care of patients, it is the doctor's duty to learn more about the disease and of those whom it afflicts. A superficial or outdated knowledge is inadequate in most branches of medicine but especially so in oncology.

SPECIFIC FACTORS

We must now consider some special factors which may influence the doctor's attitudes with the result that he approaches the cancer patient in a way that is different to that of others.

The Patient's Personality

We cannot escape the possibility that cancer may be associated with constitutional factors. Galen suggested that the temperament described by Aristotle (384–322 BC) – melancholic – was frequently associated with cancer. W. H. Walshe (*The Nature and Treatment of Cancer*, 1846) claimed that: 'Women of high colour and sanguinous temperament were more subject to mammary cancer than those of different constitutions.' H. J. Eysenck, in *Smoking, Health and Personality* (1963), reaches three conclusions: firstly, that there has been little medical interest in such possibilities; secondly, that the evidence so far available suggests that constitutional factors in general and personality factors in particular are associated with a tendency to develop cancer; and thirdly, that it would be unscientific to read too much into the work already done and that there is need for more research.

Most clincial oncologists can recall patients whose disease has apparently been under control for some time but where stress, trauma, or psychological strain have appeared to break down that control. For example, an elderly lady who had been apparently free from disease for nine years after treatment for a cancer of the breast lost her husband and only daughter in a motor car accident; within two months the chest wall was covered with secondary deposits. Again, a woman of thirty-five, free from disease for five years after treatment for an early breast cancer, also developed secondaries on the chest wall within three months of her husband's unexpected death from coronary disease. So we can go on giving anecdotal examples of sudden shock. We may add also the changes in disease pattern associated with the menopause and question whether these are due to stress, hormonal changes, constitutional factors, or to combination of some or all of these aspects. Clearly, as Eysenck points out, we need to accept that psychosomatic and personality changes may have associations with both the development and the subsequent course of malignant disease and that there is an obvious need for more research.

Now, most people respond to another's personality; it is on this that we base our likes or dislikes of other individuals. Some traits or types of personality arouse our interest or sympathy, or may leave us indifferent or frankly antagonistic. If we suggest that cancer may be associated with certain personality factors these may be just the factors that stimulate a reactionary response in certain clinicians; thus we may postulate that there exists an attitude response between patient and doctor which may be unalterable on the patient's side.

The Doctor's Response to his Patient

It is possible that the doctor's attitude may be influenced by certain aspects of the disease; for example, the type of growth, the site in the body, the extent of the malignant process, the histology, the presence of other disease processes, the co-existence of factors which may limit the patient's expectation of life. To these must be added such indefinable factors as the patient's usefulness, a young father with family responsibilities, or a young mother, or an old patient tired and ready for his life to end, beset by worries and more afraid of being kept alive than fearing to die. Even further he may be influenced by the patient's own enthusiasm, his desire to live, to help, to take his place in the community. The hypochondriac may be at a disadvantage, he is a source of worry, even irritation, to the busy doctor if past history has often shown no organic disease; thus, the investigation of new symptoms may be deferred. The doctor may pander to the apprehensive patient and agree with him that referral and treatment may be postponed; this may be no more than a desire to please but may be tempered by the doctor's own suspicion that treatment is ineffectual or that in this case the lesion is slow-growing and that a little delay is unlikely to affect the final outcome. Now we know full well that the doctor treats the patient to the best of his ability, making no difference between any, but when a decision has to be made we cannot assess how much such factors as those given may unconsciously affect the practitioner's attitude.

In recent years we hear the word 'emotion' used with derision, the implication being that the balanced, well-adjusted person does not display any emotive feeling. This is a cold approach adopted often by administrators in the health service who deal with illness from a distance, safely behind their desks objectively looking at mere statistics and reports. But medicine is not practised in this way, it is a personal service in which the practitioner cannot avoid being involved with those who suffer. Emotions cannot be swept aside, and it is difficult at times to be objective and dispassionate. Cancer produces its own emotive responses in patient, relative, friend, and medical practitioner.

Children

Whilst most clinicians will accept cancer as a disease in old people, its presence in children is accompanied with a tragic feeling of frustration and despair. The change in the pattern of child and infant mortality from that of the last century has turned what was a common occurrence into almost a rarity; indeed, the significance of a child's death has been enhanced. Because we do not expect death at this age, there is a feeling that all deaths can be and should be avoided, that it is the duty of the doctor to keep the young alive, and that someone has failed if this is not so. Next to accidents, cancer is the commonest cause of death in children under the age of fifteen.

Malignant disease occurring in childhood may be of two types: firstly, tumours found almost exclusively in children, the embryonal types such as nephroblastomas, neuroblastomas, meduloblastomas, retinoblastomas, and secondly, the childhood manifestations of those tumours found in all age groups but much more commonly found in older people.

There are problems of diagnosis, treatment, and aftercare, and because the lesion at this age is rare few clinicians have had great experience of dealing with such tumours. The diagnosis of the disease may be delayed until quite a late stage because the child is unable to communicate symptoms to the parent. The signs of disease, such as fretfulness, anorexia, and listlessness, are also those of many childhood ailments so the parent frequently delays seeking medical advice and definitive diagnosis may be made only by the exclusion of other commoner diseases. Treatment may present distinct problems, surgery may produce permanent sequelae, radiation may produce stunting of growth and even iatrogenic effects in a child who otherwise has a normal life expectancy. The social problems may be considerable; is it better for the child to be admitted to hospital for treatment? Into a paediatric ward or to a special ward associated with particular care, for example, radiotherapy? Should the mother be admitted also? If the mother is admitted what are the possible effects on the rest of the family, the husband and other siblings? How much should brothers and sisters be told? What are the likely effects of death on the family? Who will support the family? So we can go on with the list, but in each case the problem is an individual one and there are few guides to help.

Awareness of the possibility of the disease occurring in the child will alert the doctor to possible diagnosis. It is essential, however, that there is close co-operation between all the medical staff concerned with diagnosis and treatment, and the formation of paediatric oncological units is to be encouraged.

The Handicapped

Any treatment aimed at curing cancer requires that very active measures are taken. Radical treatment can only be carried out in a patient who is in reasonably good health and who is able to withstand an extensive operation or an exhaustive course of therapy by radiation or cytotoxic agents. Severe constitutional diseases may limit the extent of the therapy and it is possible that indeed such extensive therapy may accelerate the process of the constitutional disease, reduce the patient's general resistance, and shorten his life. Nothing will be achieved in giving an exhaustive course of therapy to a patient who is obviously dying, be it from his cancer or another disease: it will only make his last few days miserable. In assessing the patient's suitability for radical treatment the doctor must also take into account possible sequelae; these may leave the patient in an even worse state if he is already handicapped by disease. One must question whether much radical treatment is justifiable if it merely extends the patient's life for a few days or leaves him seriously crippled or in pain or distress. The clinician obviously must balance possible survival against quality of life when making a decision about treatment. When we consider palliation we make sure that only the minimal treatment to produce relief of symptoms is given and there is no justification for long-protracted treatment with possible sequelae.

The Elderly

Whilst age alone is not a bar to radical treatment, advanced years are often associated with a general deterioration of bodily functions and frequently with associated disease. The possibility of giving radical treatment in very elderly patients needs very careful consideration. The tissues of the elderly may not withstand high doses of radiation and may show poor healing and repair after surgery or radiotherapy. The ability of the patient to cope with sequelae such as amputation, colostomy, tracheostomy, and so on, needs careful assessment especially if there is only a small possibility of permanent cure.

The Extent of the Disease

Heroic attempts at curing an advanced disease are frequently misguided; the heroism is more correctly applied to the patient than to the doctor or the surgical procedure. There can be little justification in carrying out extensive local surgery or radiation in a patient in whom the disease has already widely disseminated and yet it is sometimes done.

Pregnancy

The patient with malignant disease who is pregnant raises particular problems for the doctor. In his response he may be influenced by several factors, his own religious beliefs about abortion, the parents' wishes and their desire to have a child, which may be influenced by the impossibility of further pregnancy either because the method of treatment may preclude this, because of the influence of a subsequent pregnancy on the course of the disease, or because the age of the patient will not allow it.

Economics

It is only in Utopia that crime, injustice, poverty, and other ills do not exist – but this exists *nowhere* and regrettably modern society is severely limited by economic considerations. Whilst we may have the world's finest Health Service it is only as good as the finances available, and there are certain restrictions. Thus, in recent years we are aware of 'cost effectiveness' and money must be spent to achieve the greatest good; it is inevitable that service needs must come before teaching and research and development. But even in the service field there are restrictions and we must decide where money can be used to the greatest advantage, where it will achieve the greatest number of cures, return the larger number of patients back to useful productive life, or ease the greatest amount of distress. The prevailing attitudes to cancer – a hopeless disease – results in less than adequate money being available. Decisions about financial allocations are inevitably made by administrators who have little personal knowledge and are reluctant to take a specialist's advice because they consider it biased – invariably they react by not spending money on the hopeless; it would be 'throwing money away'. The result is that insufficient is being allocated to this branch of medicine. An inadequate number of beds means that a doctor must decide which of his patients on a waiting list is to be admitted for a chance of a cure, and whose treatment is to be deferred; expensive apparatus becomes obsolete and breakdown causes a major financial crisis; development and research are restricted; financial inducements from overseas result in a serious depletion of trained staff. Thus we enter a vicious spiral of problems; inadequate finances means insufficient staff, beds, apparatus, and results in delay in treatment, with poorer results of therapy, a worsening public attitude to the disease resulting in the belief that money should not be spent on a hopeless disease, and so on. Such a spiral will only be broken by a reassessment of financial allocations activated by the knowledge that cancer can be cured, even prevented, and merits greater consideration than we have previously given to it if it is to be conquered.

When we consider the doctor's approach it is not possible to be dogmatic; clearly we cannot make rules or suggest possible courses of action when there are so many factors which may affect his attitude to the treatment of his patient. Often he is unaware of these factors as separate points when he makes up his mind about management. Perhaps he will benefit from consciously asking himself why he considers a certain treatment policy the best for that patient, and in this way he may be helped to balance the factors leading to his decision.

3
Attitudes to the Causes and Diagnosis of Cancer

We must now consider the doctor's attitude to the various aspects of the disease process, including such relatively theoretical studies as epidemiology, aetiology, and pathology, as well as the more clinically orientated parts, such as diagnosis, treatment, and subsequent patient care. It is inevitable that the individual clinician will be more concerned and interested in some parts more than others but his overall response shapes his subsequent approach.

Aetiology and Prevention

The early interpretations of disease were tied up with religion and magic and the belief that illness was sent by the Gods, probably as a result of wrongdoing. Aristotle (384–322 BC) initiated the study of disease processes when he propounded his four stages: firstly, the material cause of the thing, secondly, the law according to which it develops, thirdly, the starting point of the process, and, finally, the completed result.

Galen explained all diseases as resulting from one of four humours, phlegm, blood, choler, and black bile; health consisted of a balance of these and an excess of one resulted in disease; black bile was held to be responsible for cancer. His teachings had a profound effect on medical thinking for many years and it was customary to quote his causes of disease rather than to seek for any other explanation. The acceptance of previous teachings, especially if they could be construed as the will of God, fitted in with medieval life when few people had even the rudiments of education and the only ones with any learning were the clergy. So powerful was the influence of Galen on medical thought that his four humours persist today in *phlegmatic*, *sanguine*, *choleric*, and *melancholic*.

It is only in the past two centuries that doctors have searched for specific causes of disease. Epidemiology, the study of disease in the community, was perhaps not as closely linked with clinical medicine as it should have been; the clinician deals with the care of the patient with an established disease, and the epidemiologist is more concerned with the study of that disease in a group or community. Aetiology, a study of the causes, is confused by the long latent period between cause and effect ranging from about three years in the case of arsenical skin cancer, to sixty-nine years in scrotal cancer and seventy-five years in skin cancer caused by mineral oil. Such long periods raise doubts as to whether the effect is really related to the cause. Inevitably the clinician demands 'proof' and is not impressed by mere supposition or even by supportive evidence, especially when long established habits or procedures are being incriminated.

The average doctor's approach to aetiological causes is well exemplified by his reaction to cancer of the lung and cigarette smoking. Physicians have argued since tobacco was first introduced into Europe, one group extolling the virtues of tobacco as a cure for most diseases at one time or another, and the other counterbalancing by pointing out that the habit was harmful. Factual scientific evidence has now been produced to establish that smoking is in fact the causal factor in many lung cancers. One would now expect universal agreement by all doctors but there is nothing of the kind. We have developed three differing attitudes: a group of doctors who accept the facts, a group who completely reject the facts and propose alternative theories, not facts, plausible only to themselves, and a third group who believe the facts, induce their patients to stop smoking, but continue to do so themselves. An amazing group this, presenting the age-old maxim: 'Do as I say, not as I do'. If the doctor prevaricates and does not take a sufficiently firm attitude in warning of the dangers the public are confused and, taking the easy way out, continue to smoke. As a result there has been little, if any, reduction in tobacco consumption. The doctor must accept a share of responsibility in this because he has not adopted the correct attitude based on the factual medical knowledge presented to him.

Many cancers of the lung, upper respiratory tract, and bladder would be prevented if smoking was stopped; we can therefore say that these cancers are preventable. We know now that cancer of the neck of the womb, the cervix, could rightly be called a sexually transmitted disease because of its association with intercourse and that certain changes in sexual morals and hygiene could prevent it. We know the causes of many other cancers and work is actively in progress on the aetiological investigation of others. Though we may have no doubt about the importance of the causative agent in our own mind it may be difficult for us to persuade others. If the public are to benefit from the results of epidemiological investigations and the demonstration of causative aetiological factors, the clinician, who has a relationship with the general public which the epidemiologist does not have, must keep abreast of such surveys. He must develop an alertness to possible aetiological factors, must read more fully, and must co-operate more with the cancer epidemiologist.

Early Diagnosis and Detection

'Early diagnosis' implies that the patient has symptoms which need to be investigated and 'detection' that regular examinations are made with the possibility of finding occult malignant disease before symptoms occur. Such detection techniques include vaginal smears, sputum, gastric washings and urine cytology, and mass miniature radiography. These examinations may be made at 'well-person clinics'. Patients attending these clinics may indeed be well but they may have symptoms which to them appear insignificant and which they did not want to trouble their doctor with, or they may be suspicious of some unexplained symptom. They may come for reassurance because they have read of the value of such tests, or have a friend or relative who has developed cancer, or because some famous personality has the disease, or simply because they have an anxiety about malignancy. Examination may show no abnormality, suggest that further investigation is necessary or may detect an early malignancy.

The mass miniature radiography (MMR) service was very successful in detecting tuberculosis in this country and regular attendance every six to twelve months was a satisfactory method of detecting relatively early cases of the disease. However, the results with carcinoma of the bronchus have not been so rewarding. A patient may have an X-ray, be told that it shows no abnormality, be requested to report again in six months' time, but he may not do so because chest symptoms may develop, a diagnosis of cancer be made, and death result within that period. Furthermore, because his chest radiograph has been reported normal and he has been reassured that there is no chest disease, he may neglect to see his own doctor if, subsequently, chest symptoms do occur, or indeed these symptoms may be dismissed by his doctor because of the recent negative films. We may say that MMR has not made a drastic effect on the diagnosis of cancer.

Self-examination of the breast can be demonstrated to the patient who should carry it out regularly and report any suspicious findings to her own doctor. Such instruction can be given at a cancer information centre, by educational programmes, in articles in ladies' journals, or by the patient's own doctor.

The patient may have heard of methods of detection and approach her doctor for advice about attending such a clinic. This, of course, implies that the doctor has knowledge not only of the nature of the test or examination, but of where it can be carried out, and of the kind of information the patient may be given. Sometimes there may be a lack of communication between medical and lay educators. The doctor must be willing to help his inquiring patient by giving advice and encouragement. However, not all doctors are convinced about the use of such detection methods and some are genuinely concerned that patients may develop an inordinate interest amounting to a phobia or fear about the disease as a result of such widespread advertisement. By word or expression it is possible that he many reveal his criticism of methods of detection. The patient who knows her doctor may fear his ridicule at her request for such examination; this does little to set her mind at rest and consequently she may hesitate about seeking advice when she has definite symptoms.

Curative methods of treatment rely on the disease being confined to a localized area which can be removed by excision or destroyed by radiation; dissemination results in a worsening of the prognosis with little chance of cure. The first indication of malignant disease may be a rather insignificant symptom and the over-suspicious doctor could cause alarm if he immediately suspected the worst in all patients with such symptoms. Therefore he may wait for more positive evidence but this could cause delay in instituting definitive treatment. It is difficult to define an attitude of alertness which will successfully pick out those patients with malignant disease at the earliest possible moment. The increasing incidence of malignant diseases must increase the doctor's awareness of the possibility of malignancy. At one time it was more usual to take the view that malignancy was diagnosed by elimination of other diseases. Now, however, more often an attitude of suspicion eliminates the more serious disease first. This attitude at least helps to reduce delay during which distant spread could occur. The patient who is already diagnosed as having a non-malignant condition poses a problem; small changes in symptoms and signs may be mistaken for progression of the disease. For example, a patient with chronic bronchitis may have blood in his sputum which could be benign in origin or could indicate the presence of co-existent malignant disease. The persistently anxious patient who is always attending with a new symptom is a difficult problem; many times there is no reason for alarm, but remember Aesop's shepherd boy who cried 'wolf'. The doctor thus has to develop an attitude of alertness to suspicious details together with a knowledge of early signs and symptoms and of methods of detection. As soon as definite symptoms or signs develop he must not hesitate to investigate further.

Pathology

The importance of histological confirmation of the clinical diagnosis of malignant disease needs no emphasis. Although the clinical diagnosis is correct in a large proportion of cases, only microscopical examination of a piece of tissue will give a true indication of the nature of the tumour. The desire to confirm the diagnosis, however, produces two conflicting attitudes regarding management. On the one hand we have the desire to obtain a positive diagnosis before treatment is started, which is counteracted with a desire to disturb the tissues as little as possible so as to prevent dissemination. Manipulation of any tumour may possibly cause spread and this may lead to a reluctance to perform an operation. Surgical operations will open up venous and lymphatic channels and it is theoretically possible that the smaller the incision into the growth, the less chance there is of metastasis; thus needle biopsy has attained some popularity in recent years.

Insistence on obtaining positive histological evidence may result in delay in starting treatment whilst many investigations are carried out; clearly the clinician's insistence on perfection may be to the patient's disadvantage, especially in rapidly growing tumours. A balance therefore must be struck between the desire for positive histological proof and an acceptance of the clinical diagnosis if proof cannot be obtained quickly.

It is very desirable to be certain of the whole clinical picture before proceeding to surgical operation if it is at all possible; the patient then knows what is to happen to him and so do the surgical team, the ward, and the relatives. For example, some clinicians will carry out a biopsy using a needle or small drill in a breast tumour; this is a minor procedure performed in outpatients and a pathological report is made within twenty-four hours. When the patient is admitted, she can then be informed of the need for removal of the breast and the whole surgical team know the full nature of the operation to be undertaken. Compare this with the alternative of an operation to remove a piece of tissue, urgent histological examination proceeding to removal if indicated; the patient is anaesthetized and does not know whether she will wake up with her breast removed or not, the operating theatre staff, the ward staff, and the relatives are not sure of the nature of the operation until the pathological report is available.

Most biopsies are of a relatively minor nature and are often performed under local anaesthetic. The patient, even though he may not have a true knowledge of the possible nature of the disease, views the biopsy as a major point in his care; on it depends the whole of his future treatment. It is surprising how many patients sense this and dread the need for biopsy and fear to know the result.

Although histological proof of malignancy is always desirable, every attempt should be made to obtain this by the quickest possible method. If this is not possible and if there is likely to be delay which may jeopardize the prognosis the clinician must rely on his clinical diagnosis and proceed to give treatment without positive pathological proof in some cases.

DOUBLE PRIMARIES

There is a very popular attitude that insists that all symptoms should, if possible, be associated with one disease and indeed very frequently they can be. In malignant disease it is not unusual to find that whatever symptom the patient subsequently develops it is originally thought to be a further spread of the malignant process. Once a patient has been to a radiotherapy department he is frequently referred back with any new symptoms. Now, of course, these could be due to a non-malignant process and it is a reflection on our non-acceptance of the possibility of *cure* that suggests that they are malignant. Investigation of all subsequent symptoms is essential and it is better that recurrence is initially suspected and treated, if necessary, and then if it is excluded a start can be made on treatment for the less serious condition.

The possibility of a second primary growth should always be kept in mind because:

1. The same causative agent may be acting on the same soil; for example, skin carcinomas may be multiple in oil workers; a patient who has been a heavy smoker may be cured of one lung cancer and develop another; a patient who has had a mastectomy for cancer of the breast may develop one on the other side.

2. The same causative agent may affect different organs – one of the commonest double primary combinations is cancer of the lung and bladder, both due to smoking tobacco.

3. It is possible that some patients have an inherent, possibly inherited, susceptibility to develop a malignant disease either *de novo* or as a result of some stimulus; or alternatively that they have no resistance to the effect of such a stimulus. Such people may develop two or more malignancies at different sites suggesting that there is a common causative agent.

Thus 'once bitten, twice shy', the patient who has had a malignant disease is carefully watched and indeed a second primary may be discovered earlier because of this. If the lesion is a new primary it could be cured, but if it is a secondary deposit this is inevitably part of a widespread dissemination with a poor prognosis. It is important, therefore, to determine which it is and not to adopt an attitude which accepts that it is spread and nothing can be done for it.

4

Attitudes to the Treatment of Cancer

The attitudes to treatment may affect the clinician's approach to the disease.

Surgery

It is almost a basic concept that if a thing is diseased it should be removed; this is our approach in horticulture to rot and decay, to pollution – natural then that if an organ or part thereof in the body is diseased it should be removed.

Provided the tumour has not attached itself to vital structures or extended beyond the surgical limits, a cure would appear possible. Improvements in surgical and anaesthetic techniques have made it possible to carry out complex procedures to remove the primary tumour and possible involved lymph nodes, and if necessary to perform plastic or repair operations. In his basic training the doctor obtains a good idea of the efficacy of operations and the expected complications and he can then advise his patient and the relatives. The general practitioner frequently gives this preliminary advice to the patient before referring him to hospital. Such advice given by a friend or well-known acquaintance – and that is the role that the general practitioner frequently plays – is far more valuable than that of the hospital doctor whom the patient meets for the first time, in unfamiliar circumstances, and of whom, because the nature of his illness creates anxiety, fear, and worry, he stands in some awe. We must remember that the patient frequently is worried about the need for treatment and the remote possibility that a serious operation may be necessary, and that in his own mind he has also nursed the possibility that he may have a cancer and that it is hopeless. Education of the medical student and young doctor in surgery and surgical techniques is therefore of immense importance.

In considering surgical procedures the clinician will take into account the suitability of the patient for operation, including his general condition, the extent of the tumour and the type of operation, the morbidity, the possible complications, and the effect that these will have on the patient's future life and work.

The theory behind surgery for cancer has always been that of total removal of the tumour and cure, and a series of operations may be required to achieve this. For many years nothing or very little was offered to the inoperable patient, but recently palliative surgery has achieved some success in relieving him of distressing symptoms, as for example short circuit operations on the bowel, insertion of a tube into the oesophagus or stomach, a transplant of ureters, and toilet surgery for fungating offensive tumours.

In very recent years a new phrase has come into use, 'preventive cancer surgery', aimed at removing those lesions which have a propensity for malignant change; such lesions include keratoses, post-radiation dermatitis, leucoplakia, gastric ulcers, and intestinal polyps or thyroid nodules. It is important to establish that malignant change occurs in a proportion of these lesions. Few medical practitioners would doubt the advisability of carrying out what is often a relatively simple operation to prevent a malignant disease developing. However, we can take the argument further; what of the young patient who has had treatment for a carcinoma of the breast? The same exciting factor is presumably present and can act on the same soil of the remaining breast; what then of the suggestion to remove the second breast as a preventive measure? What of the patient who has no further use for a uterus; there is an obvious indication for hysterectomy if she has heavy periods due to uterine fibroids or if the cervix is diseased, since a possible source of cancer can be removed. But what if there is no clinical indication, is removal of a healthy organ justified then?

Recurrent tumours may require further surgery with an obviously poorer prognosis. The clinician may be hesitant to persuade a patient to undergo a further operation for a condition which has not responded to previous surgical treatment. Here he must weigh up the possibilities, if the previous operation was only just inadequate, a 'geographical miss', removal of a wider margin of tissue is obviously justified and he will have no hesitation in recommending this. More complex is the patient with advancing metastases, especially when a 'chasing technique' is used, each removal being followed by a recurrence a little further ahead. The problem is to know when to give up, and here we have to balance the eventual outcome against the surgical trauma and mental distress; too frequently the disease is out of control and the patient ends his life with the stress of recurrent operations leading to the realization of the hopelessness of his condition.

Very extensive operations, sometimes called 'heroic surgery', call for particular consideration; fortunately these are now being replaced with improvements in and greater realization of the possibilities of radiotherapy.

There is no place for 'disciplinary pride'; because a patient is initially referred to a surgeon does not mean that the only treatment is surgery. There is little doubt that this was once a mistaken medical attitude but the patient needs the best treatment, and should be referred to the appropriate specialist for this. The experience gained at combined surgical and radiotherapeutic clinics has helped to achieve greater collaboration. It is to be hoped that our prevailing interest in oncology will even further help to determine the optimal treatment conditions for each type of cancer.

Surgery is such a well-established specialty that there is little that influences the doctor's personal attitude to it. He may feel the hopelessness of carrying out a surgical procedure if there is only a small chance of success especially if the patient is likely to be severely handicapped or has widespread disease. He may question the advisability of procedures which only prolong life without curing or palliating. He may resist attempts at heroic surgery. On the other hand he may feel very strongly, in spite of his clinical experience, that 'while there is life there is hope', and that until an attempt is made to remove a lesion he cannot be sure of its inoperability. This, of course, underlies the practice of exploratory operations. But he bases his attitude on a considerable knowledge and experience which began in his undergraduate training, he is seldom suspicious of the surgeon's advice and is usually prepared to accept that decision.

We now turn to two other methods of treatment which do not enjoy the same respect and acceptance.

Radiotherapy

The practice of radiotherapy was developed by a complex system of trial and error and inevitably bad effects or complications were remembered. The reactions on the skin were at times quite severe, dry desquamation leading to moist desquamation, universally referred to as radiation 'burns' and accepted as an overdose effect due to misuse of radiation or to radiation being inexpertly applied. It was unfortunate that this treatment was expected to produce an effect which caused suffering and concern both to the patient and to his practitioner. The absorption of energy in the tissues and the formation of breakdown tissue products resulted in the radiation 'sickness' which caused the patient distress and, in the days before anti-emetic agents, exercised the doctor's skill to devise diets and conditions to reduce suffering.

Radiotherapy came into a new era with the development of super-voltage machines in the early 1950s. Sophisticated radiation techniques have resulted in better treatment, fewer untoward reactions, and a higher dose on the tumour with lower doses on surrounding normal tissues. In addition special techniques have been developed for irradiation at particular sites. Controlled clinical trials have enabled us to determine the optimal treatment conditions for certain cancers. Radiotherapy has now become a complex medical specialty requiring co-operation with all branches of medicine, with biologists and physicists and with many other disciplines.

We must examine the doctor's approach to radiotherapy and again an attempt will be made to pick out the factors which influence this. These are:

IGNORANCE

Radiotherapy is essentially a post-graduate subject, and is not taught as such to undergraduates. In the attempt to protect the medical student from the scientific complexities of radiotherapy, including physics, statistics, radiobiology, and other scientific aspects, the whole subject and its place in the treatment of malignant disease has been largely omitted. Fortunately some advance has been made and in many medical schools a few lectures are given, but too frequently by a surgeon, a physician, or even a pathologist. In a few more enlightened centres a course of lectures is given by a radiotherapist followed by visits to the radiotherapy wards and, in a very few centres students attend for elective periods. Radiotherapy is not an academic subject in many medical schools and it is somewhat the Cinderella of medicine in the eyes of many other hospital specialties. Unfortunately this attitude probably accounts for the poor recruitment of suitable doctors into the speciality.

SUSPICION

There is little doubt that the average doctor has some misgivings about a qualified doctor who takes up physics, mathematics, statistics, and certain aspects of science, subjects which once appeared to be stumbling blocks at an early time in his own career. No wonder then that the radiotherapist is looked upon as a scientist or technician and not always as a clinician who uses this extra knowledge to improve his patients' care. These subjects hold some mystique which the clinician cannot appreciate so he doubts the method of treatment. The radiotherapist is largely to blame for this attitude; he has become somewhat isolated from his fellow clinicians because of his special scientific interests.

EXPERIENCE

The clinician may have had poor results from the treatment of patients he has referred for radiotherapy. This may have arisen because the radiotherapist has not been sufficiently critical in his selection of patients for treatment and has treated advanced dying patients with little hope of cure, or has treated otherwise unsuitable patients, perhaps because of his desire to please the referring clinician. The result is that the referring doctor eventually believes that radiotherapy does no good. All the patients he has had treated have done badly, hence it follows that radiotherapy is bad. Eventually he will not refer patients until they are in a terminal stage of the disease.

PALLIATION

There is a popular belief that radiotherapy should only be given as a palliative procedure, therefore treatment is delayed until symptoms which need palliation arise and radical treatment is no longer possible. Again, there is a belief that the results of radiotherapy do not justify the mental trauma caused to the patient by referring him for this treatment. This is a somewhat unusual approach which is by no means uncommon. When the patient's condition deteriorates sufficiently to require palliation, and even the patient and his relatives are fully aware of the hopelessness of the condition, the referring clinician has no hesitation in sending the patient.

DISBELIEF

Statistical reports produced by radiotherapists may not be believed by many practitioners; there is a suspicion that the radiotherapist produces these to boost his morale and that of his staff. Of course, if the doctor has had no experience of radiotherapy, or has been taught that its use is palliative only, the production of any rate of survival can cause him so much surprise that he is likely to think it is the result of special selection or is fabricated.

We can conclude that the chief reason for these attitudes to radiotherapy stems from a lack of knowledge and inexperience.

Chemotherapy

Mysterious invisible rays may not be completely acceptable whereas drugs are more easily accepted.

The drugs used are toxic to growing cells and thus can be used when the tumour has disseminated widely throughout the body. They will, of course, affect all living cells, especially such sensitive tissues as the bone marrow; the dose of drugs that can be given thus depends on the effect they have on the blood count and only very sensitive tumours will respond. However, such drugs have caused marked improvements in the therapy of some rapidly growing tumours to the extent that we are now talking of long remission, survivors for many years, and even cures. These drugs have produced dramatic results in the leukaemias and in some other less common diseases. They will also cause some regression of the tumour, often to a marked degree, and are used to palliate the patient who is troubled by widespread metastases. Such drugs may also be used to improve the results of treatment by surgical removal and radiotherapy. There are many drugs available and some are more efficacious than others for certain diseases; combinations of certain drugs have also been investigated and in this way we can often enhance the effect of the drugs producing less toxic effects on the normal tissues. There is a need for considerable research to determine what drugs used either singly or in combination give the best result and also to determine whether the established results of treatment by surgery or radiotherapy can be improved by adjuvant radiotherapy.

The idea of using drugs has always appealed to all concerned with cancer because it suggests that with development we could produce a drug to cure all cancers; but cancer is a very mixed group of malignant diseases extending from very sensitive to very resistant types of growth, and whilst the more sensitive ones have shown a good response there appears to be little hope that the others will also respond.

In some centres it appears that chemotherapeutic agents are considered a panacea for all malignancies, and it is interesting to note such statements as 'vast improvement', 'satisfactory results', 'unexpected responses', applied where statistical results giving survival rates for a period of years are virtually unknown. Heroic attempts to cure a patient riddled with malignant disease may be justified if there is a reasonable chance of cure but not if such treatment only adds to his terminal misery, nausea, toxic effects, hair loss, and so on.

Although many hospital doctors are quite willing to assume responsibility for chemotherapy techniques, even without preliminary experience, it is commendable to note that the vast majority of family doctors consider that such therapy requires careful control with haematological examinations and leave it to the specialist.

Hormonal Therapy

The application of hormonal agents follows very much the same argument. All doctors are aware of the changes in the body due to hormones and any doctor can administer these drugs with little or no previous experience. Again the control of such drugs and a clear indication that they should be administered in a rational way is appreciated by the vast majority of family doctors. There is no place for indiscriminate experimentation with either hormones or cytotoxic agents, and all information obtained must be recorded carefully and analysed in an attempt to determine the optimal treatment conditions for a particular disease.

Immunotherapy

At the moment there is little more than an optimistic hope that this form of treatment will work, and much research work needs to be done before definite attitudes to therapy can be established.

Unproven Methods of Treatment

It is a natural tendency to view all treatments that do not conform with current thinking with a certain scepticism. This has always been so in medicine, the new or unproved treatment being suspect, but the very need for such attempts at cure arises because there is no recognized method of treatment which produces a degree of success. We are well aware that some well-known folk remedies used by country people have eventually been proved to have active principles, and so any treatment which claims to help the patient must be adequately investigated by a responsible body, but it is not uncommon to find that many so-called tumours have had no pathological confirmation. Public opinion will demand that unfortunate victims are not exploited by charlatans and quacks, who unfortunately have always been with us. The only positive way of excluding their work is to improve public education and attempt to provide better treatment.

Many of these unproven methods result from an urgent desire to produce an effective agent against all malignant diseases. Frequently they are nothing more than 'shots in the dark' often unsupported by basic medical or physiological principles. At times there would appear to be some biochemical basis but often this is a blind addition of an element or compound to an organic ring hoping that the resultant drug will have a different effect to the original substance. In this category we may include many of the forgotten cytotoxic agents.

Clearly all new methods of treatment should be thoroughly tested before extravagant claims are made about them.

Placebo Treatment

Many doctors believe that the patient who is ill expects treatment, that even if cure is not possible or palliation necessary something must appear to be done or else the patient will feel neglected. This belief goes back to the days when the patient expected a bottle of medicine from his doctor, and indeed that belief is apparent in a few patients even today. Progress over the past century has extended the expectation of life and it is now considered that the doctor should be able to achieve this irrespective of the disease. The desire of the doctor to try and help even the incurable, to bring about 'miracles', is understandable and indeed it must be recognized that no disease really is incurable until death occurs. We must accept that inroads into the problems of incurable disease are only made as a result of trying to cure even when commonsense suggests otherwise, and medical technology has already achieved many advances which a few years ago were considered impossible.

Everyone expects more with modern medicine, there are scientific 'miracles' every day; thus the unfortunate gets transferred from one doctor to another for an opinion or is admitted to some clinic making claims but with little or no hope of being benefited by the treatment.

Clinicians need to understand when to stop; usually this comes with experience, but it is necessary to consider carefully before submitting the patient to useless attempts which may increase his terminal suffering. Chemotherapy has taken the place of radiotherapy as a placebo but it is unfortunate that some patients without hope are subjected to intensive treatment even though there is no evidence that the drug will produce more than a transitory effect, and often the side effects may sometimes be marked. We must resist giving any treatment which is aimed only at seeing what the results are likely to be.

It is hard, of course, for the clinician to develop an attitude of mind that leads him to make the correct judgement every time he is presented with a patient who has cancer. This will only be brought about as a result of his own clinical experience, and from his reading and assessment of reported research projects. The clinician responsible for therapy has three choices: radical treatment aimed at cure, palliative aimed at relief of distressing symptoms, and no treatment if there is no chance of cure and no symptoms to be relieved. Each choice requires a decision made as a result of experience and careful consideration of facts, but while the first two are active, the last is passive. It is important that the patients for whom nothing can be done do not get a feeling of hopelessness passed on from the doctor.

Assessment of Results

In many cases we look for methods of curing the lesion. For example, a hernia can be cured by operation; there is no longer a weakness of the musculature with prolapse of the bowel, and, again, pneumonia may be cured when the bacteria are killed, the symptoms are cleared, and the lung returns to normal. So we can go on giving examples. It is important to realize that many conditions in medicine are not cured but controlled; for example, diabetes, asthma, and nephritis. In cancer, however, it would be presumptuous to talk of cure; this would imply that there is not one cancer cell remaining in the body which could multiply and form a tumour mass. We are unable therefore even to talk about cure in the true sense of the word. More usually we talk about survival, that is, the number of years lived after treatment. Sometimes we like to make a division between 'alive with disease' and 'alive without disease' – this is, of course, an artificial division and indicates only that clinical examination can or cannot detect recurrent disease. The only true fact which can be ascertained is whether the patient is *alive* or *dead* – and for what period of time. Thus we adopt an index of the efficiency of treatment – the survival rate.

SURVIVAL RATES
We can express the results of treatment as the number of patients surviving after a certain period of time – this is usually five years, expressed as the *five year survival rate*. But we know that as time goes on the probability of dying in cancer patients becomes no greater than in a normal population of the same age and sex – this is called the *normal life expectancy*.

When we come to make comparisons between differing treatments there is need for mathematical analysis and for tests of statistical significance. Now the doctor treating cancer patients cannot ignore this, he is looking for improved methods of treatment and he must show that a new technique is statistically better. Thus, he can no longer take a cynical view of medical statistics, he must understand them and apply them to his work. In all his work he strives for accuracy in diagnosis, in treatment, in comparison of survival rates; however, accuracy is not absolute, it is always relative and requires statistical analysis or assessment.

A further comparison of treatments calls for an assessment of morbidity, which is made up of that from the disease, the treatment, and the complications. These are difficult subjective aspects which must be compared in some way. It is not easy to apply a mathematical assessment to these criteria – for example, consider the difficulties of trying to assess pain – this can only be done by patient responses – does it incapacitate him? Is it relieved by mild analgesics? (specify what are mild); does it need more powerful analgesics? (specify); and so on. Even when we have devised some method of assessing subjective responses we meet further problems because one patient may be able to carry out his normal work, another can only perform light work, yet another may be bedridden, yet all may have the same degree of restriction of function. We find problems because we are dealing with individuals, who all respond in their own particular way.

5
Attitudes to After-Care

After treatment the patient is seen regularly by the doctor in the out-patient clinic:

(a) To continue the care of the patient. The clinician looks for a recurrence of the malignancy, for complications or untoward reactions from treatment, and anything else for which he could give further treatment or relieve the symptoms.

(b) To reassure the patient about his general health, the course of the disease, or symptoms which may be worrying him.

(c) To record details of the patient so that he can analyse the results of treatment.

(d) To review the fitting of any appliances, to consider refashioning of colostomies, or to carry out any corrective procedures such as plastic surgery.

Few patients object to these regular visits made for examination because they are worried and look forward to being reassured. Most general practitioners recognize the importance of regular follow-up also, and this is particularly true of patients treated by radiotherapy, where reactions are familiar only to the person using a certain radiation technique and where the possibility of further treatment can only be assessed by the therapist.

Follow-up clinics are time-consuming and sometimes the patient may question their need or usefulness; some patients refuse to attend, some delay seeking further advice even though they realize that all is not going well, perhaps from a fear of further treatment or of being told that nothing further can be done. In some conditions it may be quite clear to the doctor that nothing more can be done, but it would be cruel to suggest that further attendance is unnecessary, it is the final intimation of hopelessness. In other conditions it is clearly important to see the patient regularly, especially if further treatment can be given should recurrence occur. For example, if radiotherapy fails to cure an early carcinoma of the larynx radical operation may still cure.

It is usual to hold follow-up clinics at the centre where treatment has been given, so that further treatment can be given if necessary. Although it would be very desirable for the consultant to hold clinics in consultation with the family doctor, this is usually impracticable because the number of malignant cases in any one practice is likely to be small and there are insufficient consultants; there is an obvious need, however, for closer co-operation between family doctor and consultant and we must look for ways to bring this about.

The most important aspect of follow-up is to create the right atmosphere or relationship between doctor – usually specialist – and patient. The patient benefits because he knows that he can receive expert help and advice as soon as he requires it. That this attitude is achieved is evidenced by the high percentage of patients who attend or seek a further appointment if a visit is missed.

Rehabilitation

The clinician should be concerned in all aspects of patient care including the rehabilitation.

We believe that the restoration of normal or near normal capacities will become increasingly important during the next decade so that the need for rehabilitation is urgent. It is a problem which must be tackled now.

(Foreword, *Rehabilitation. Report of a Sub-Committee of the Standing Medical Advisory Committee.* Her Majesty's Stationery Office 1972.)

This report on rehabilitation is a reflection of our present thinking, that, whereas some years ago rehabilitation was considered only in patients who had received injuries, had undergone amputation of a limb, or were paralysed, crippled, or arthritic, we are concerned now also with the rehabilitation of people suffering from many diseases, the elderly, psychiatric patients, alcoholics, and drug addicts. Attempts are being made to restore people back to a level of health and activity where they can be absorbed back into the community. The report was very welcome; at last we were making an active attempt at restoring our sick to health and strength. Alas, it was not as encouraging as it would appear; whilst almost every disease is mentioned we find only one brief reference to the cancer patient: 'From time to time requests are made for special facilities for groups of patients; for example, those suffering from cancer or tuberculosis' (para. 241). The rehabilitation of the cancer patient would seem to demand as much attention as that of any other disease, but the current attitude to malignant diseases results in requests for rehabilitation being made only 'from time to time'. The possible reasons are:

(a) The concept of rehabilitating the cancer patient is somewhat novel; whilst much medical activity is devoted to the diagnosis, cure, and palliation of malignant disease we certainly have not given the same attention to returning the afflicted patient to active life.

(b) The profound pessimism which is so widely felt when cancer is diagnosed results in our having to convince our medical colleagues, nurses, ancillary workers, health administrators, and charitable bodies that rehabilitation is even to be considered in this disease.

(c) The responsibility for the rehabilitation of cancer patients has never been clearly apportioned; should it be the surgeon, the radiotherapist, the rehabilitation unit if there is one, the rheumatologist, or the general practitioner? Clearly it involves the co-operation of many people, in the hospital and in the community.

Cure of malignant disease is possible in a number of patients; many have no lasting disfigurement or complication, but some have a permanent morbidity which prevents them from carrying out their previous occupation and may need retraining to undertake lighter work.

Even if treatment is unsuccessful in achieving a cure, the disease may be controlled to such an extent that the patient may have several months, or even years, of relatively normal life. It is important that this time is spent to the fullest, that he and his family make the most of what time is left, and that he maintains, if at all possible, his dignity as a working man providing for his family.

When there are inadequate facilities or finance for any rehabilitation service it is small wonder that the 'hopeless disease' is pushed to the end of the queue. Obviously we must re-assess our priorities and in keeping with current attitudes to rehabilitation we must demand adequate facilities for cancer patients. We need to change the current medical attitude to one which accepts retraining and rehabilitation in the patient who has had a malignant disease.

6

Attitudes to Pain and Suffering

We are all of us predestined to pain. It is in pain that our mother gives birth to us; it is pain which heralds our entrance into the world. It is pain which is everywhere around us on earth. Why does pain exist? We shall see that it is to religion that we must look for consolation in suffering; and that not only suffering is our inevitable lot upon earth, but that it is for our advantage to have to undergo pain and suffering. The subject is not only one of full importance but it is one of immense comfort to us all.

(Agostino da Monte Jelro, *Pain*, 1887)

It has long been considered that pain, a necessary attribute of man, was associated with sin and da Monte Jelro goes further to suggest that this was passed on to us because of the original sin in the Garden of Eden when Adam and Eve abused their freedom. The three guilty ones shared the punishment, the serpent to crawl upon its belly, the woman in sorrow to bring forth her children, and the man to have sorrow all the days of his life with the promise that he would return as dust to the ground which provided him with food. This is the thought that has filled man from early days, that disobedience caused suffering, woe, and pain; we find many references in literature to this idea which have enjoined us to accept that suffering and pain are the fruits of misbehaviour and sin. This attitude is not solely found in history or even among untutored or uncivilized people or races. It is prevalent in our modern thinking and is frequently reiterated in a somewhat oblique way by our patients today. 'But why have I developed this, doctor? I have always lived a clean/healthy/good/blameless life – I cannot think what I have done to deserve this.' The implication is that the disease/pain/suffering is a consequence upon some sin – perhaps rightly deserved – a punishment. I have no doubt that this reasoning goes on in the minds of many of our patients with malignant disease. Perhaps it was more frequent some years ago when we saw more cases of malignancy developing upon syphilitic ulcers, when the cause and effect were more obvious to the patient. Today there still remains a desire to find an aetiological factor and sin – in all its forms – fits easily into this category in many people's minds.

The belief that pain is sent from God does of course, produce a paradox: 'How can a God who is devoted to love, to helping, to forgiveness and so on, inflict pain on those he loves?' Religious faith suggests that pain is only a testing reaction sent to prove the worth of the individual, to strengthen his character, to make him appreciate his God. Suffering is thought to develop character and often great things have been produced by those who have known pain and suffering; Dante (1265–1321) suffered unknown agonies when he was banished from Florence; Milton (1608–74), blinded, was to ask: 'Doth God exact day labour light deny'd?'; blind also was Handel (1685–1759), and Homer too according to tradition, and so we can go on. We remember also many great warriors who, injured in battle, often with permanent effects, have fought on to be heroes and brave leaders. Whilst death was the prerequisite of the martyr, the term 'confessor' was awarded to those who experienced suffering and pain short of death. Thus we have revered those who have suffered.

Suffering was acceptable by some tribes, signs of discomfort were abhorred, thus the pubertal rites associated with incision and scarification are borne without complaint. Bloodshed and suffering were well-known in some civilizations, for example, the Romans and their amphitheatres, the Middle Ages abound with stories of adversities and hardships, suffering and pain were almost necessities of some monastic communities. We have ample evidence then that man accepts pain and is prepared to suffer; indeed he may in some circumstances welcome the discomfort and even seek it.

Looking at pain more biologically, we appreciate that it is a warning of danger; experience of pain and the association of ideas is in fact one way of teaching the child about the dangers of its environment. Fire burns and produces pain, a knife cuts and produces pain. Pain demands investigation, thus a patient presenting with severe abdominal pain is investigated before it is relieved; if the cause is an inflamed appendix the necessary steps to relieve by removal of the inflamed organ are taken. Pain may limit movement of a limb when this would be disadvantageous; toothache warns of the need for dental care, and so we can go on. Pain is a positive symptom which cannot be ignored for long and which sends the patient to the doctor for advice.

The doctor's attitude to pain is influenced by his own emotive response and it is possible that this may affect his reaction to pain and suffering in the malignant patient. We have previously mentioned the association of ideas that may occur in people's minds, especially that cancer is synonymous with suffering and death. There is such a close association between cancer and pain and cancer and suffering that it is expected that these are prominent symptoms in this disease. Furthermore some patients with early cancer show their relief in thinking that because there is no pain the diagnosis could not possibly be that of a malignant disease. It is important that the doctor does not share this basic attitude; experience and knowledge will convince him that this is far from correct, even in the terminal stages of the disease.

Pain is essentially a subjective symptom and as such relies on individual interpretation. Even the experienced medical worker is unable to assess with any degree of accuracy the severity of a patient's pain, but he can make a rough guess when he knows the amount of analgesic necessary to bring relief. It is possible that in one individual a pain which is incapacitating may be borne without distress by another – of course I cannot in any way substantiate that statement; it is an impression only. The doctor's attitude to his patient in pain will depend on his own appreciation, his 'pain threshold', as it is sometimes called. It will depend on his tolerance to some extent, and also on his sympathy and on other factors present in his own make-up, whether he is introspective himself or the 'tough-rugged' type. Whilst he may have every sympathy for one patient, he may detect or imagine a degree of malingering or even a desire for attention and limelight in another, and this may affect his response.

The patient may complain of varying types of pain. Acute pain may be found at any time and usually suggests a serious condition such as bone involvement or pathological fracture; this is essentially a warning pain. Chronic pain is more constant in nature and more resistant to simple analgesics; this is the more usual type of pain in terminal disease. As the disease progresses the patient's will-power and resistance decrease and the pain which earlier on may have been bearable or perhaps not fully appreciated now becomes unbearable, breaking him down by its very persistence.

E. Wilkes, talking of his experience in general practice in *People and Cancer* (1969), expected about one half of the patients dying at home to have only trivial pain, twenty per cent to have bad pain for about two weeks, whereas in thirteen per cent pain was present for up to six weeks. Acute pain occurring as a result of a growing tumour is frequently alleviated by radiotherapy but analgesics may be required until relief is obtained.

We have been shown very effectively how to deal with the pain of malignant disease by workers at St Christopher's Hospice, London, St Luke's Nursing Home, Sheffield, St Joseph's Hospital, The Hostel of God, the Marie Curie Homes, and other similar organizations. As a result of their work it is now accepted that it is not a necessary concomitant, that it can be relieved in practically every case, that the patient does not need such heavy sedation that he cannot live with those around him, that pain can be relieved by giving regular small doses of analgesics even if there is no pain at the time the drug is given, that adequate control of pain demands frequent alteration of drug and dose and timing during the illness, that individual attention is of tremendous importance, and that to assess the patient's pain the doctor must take time to listen and to gain his confidence.

I do not wish to write more about the relief of pain here; excellent articles have already been written and we can safely say that many problems of pain can be controlled. Many patients can be adequately dealt with at home but a few do need hospital admission and some, because of the special nature of the pain, do need expert care such as that given in terminal homes. In spite of our ability to control pain we do still see patients who suffer. Often this is due to the ineffective use of analgesics and doctors must adopt an attitude which questions why pain is present and look for ways of relieving it. To accept that pain is inevitable is a sign of medical defeat.

Not all pain is adequately relieved by analgesics, for example, bone pain due to invasion by primary growth or metastases. There seems to be some evidence that tension in the bone plays a part because pathological fracture frequently produces relief. This pain can frequently be relieved by a short palliative course of radiation consisting of one, two, or up to five, treatments. Radiotherapy should be tried for pain due to malignant disease but if relief is not obtained the sensory nerve pathway can be disrupted by anaesthetizing the nerve or by cutting the sensory nerve tracts of the spinal cord.

So far I have deliberately confined my remarks to pain because that is foremost in most people's minds. But this is not the only cause of suffering; there are many others. Nausea and vomiting may occur, possibly due to the associated toxaemia due to the breakdown of tissues or to the effects of radiation, especially when the upper abdomen is treated; both symptoms can be relieved with anti-emetics if the clinician appreciates the cause. Bleeding from a recurrent tumour producing blood in the sputum, the vomit, the urine, faeces, and so on, can often be relieved or reduced by palliative radiation treatment. There is a popular belief that if a patient has had a course of radiotherapy further treatment cannot be given. This is usually incorrect, and should the patient have symptoms caused by residual disease he can still be given palliative therapy. We often give one or two treatments to terminal patients who suffer pain to make their last few days tolerable.

Malaise and exhaustion may be due to anaemia which should be corrected if possible. Infection is a frequent concomitant especially in lung cancer and can be relieved by large doses of antibiotics. Fear and upset may be helped by suitable tranquillizers. The patient's appetite can frequently be improved with medicines or drinks having a bitter taste, frequent small light meals being preferable to the occasional heavy feast. Emotional distress may be caused by fungating, unsightly, or offensive lesions; some healing may be achieved with appropriate treatment and at times deodorants may help. Colostomies, especially if poorly controlled, may cause unnecessary suffering when recent and because the patient thinks that he is offensive and objectionable. It is heartening to see that, with encouragement, in a very short time he is able to manage very well and takes his place in society without embarrassment.

We must remember too the emotional suffering of the man who feels he is no longer a useful member of society or who cannot conceive of the future if he cannot do the job for which he was trained. Sympathetic listening and advice may help him to forget and look forward to rehabilitation.

It becomes clear that the doctor's own attitude to suffering is an important factor; he may have been influenced in the past to strive only for radical treatment and a cure. The inability to cure the patient may be construed as a failure on his part and because treatment has failed he may, in a way, lose interest in the patient and fail to give palliative treatment aimed at relieving symptoms.

It is not always possible to assess the degree of suffering experienced by any individual patient. Whilst some will seek alleviation of only relatively minor degrees of suffering, others will endure extremes in the desire to show fortitude or in the belief that it is expected of them or helps them in some way. Experience helps us to detect these patients, and we suspect that they are in pain; we therefore seek their confidence so that they can report without embarrassment and help us to assess the effects of the drugs given. Other upsetting symptoms are more frequently spoken of and can be observed by the caring team.

There is still one further aspect of suffering to be considered; the suffering that may be caused unnecessarily to a patient in a desire to do him good. Radical treatment given in cases where there is no hope of cure may produce its own upset; we must realise that nothing will be achieved by prolonged courses of therapy given to a patient who is already doomed, and we may cause distress. Whatever our attitude to distress in the treatment of cancer let it never be said that the patient suffered many things from the physician, but rather that the doctor helped to relieve pain and suffering and helped to heal.

7
Attitudes to Terminal Care and Death – Euthanasia

Whilst medical care has been involved mainly with restoring the patient to normal health or alleviating suffering, less attention has been paid to those patients who have lost the race and are about to die; for them there is little more than tender loving care during their gradual decline. In relatively recent years homes or hospitals have been devoted especially to the care of these patients, and throughout the country groups of doctors have become specialized in their care. These doctors seek to bring about the relief of physical pain and suffering, to instil peace of mind, to alleviate mental stress and upset, and to maintain the dignity that should be associated with dying.

Doctors, nurses, and others sometimes think that the dying patient needs to be protected from everything going on around him and that noise or distraction may be upsetting to him, whereas frequently he is fully aware of these happenings and anxious to feel involved. Isolation as practised in many hospitals may not be the best for such patients; even a comatose patient may have an acute sense of hearing and touch, and the presence of another person is obvious to him. Quietness then is not always advantageous and the patient may welcome physical contact.

We must decide where the individual should be at the time of his death. It is not possible to be dogmatic; whilst the majority of people would prefer to die at home in the midst of their family, this is not always so. Some prefer to die away from the loved ones to whom they may cause distress, they may be embarrassed or upset that their family may see them in a state of distress or of incontinence. Again, it may be preferable that a patient does not die at home if, for example, he is in need of continuous analgesics or if the only person at home to look after him is elderly – remember that cancer is a disease of old age and that frequently there is only the spouse of approximately the same age who may be disabled, chronically sick, or unable to cope with the physical strain, let alone the mental and emotional stress. The home conditions may be uncongenial or over-crowded or inconvenient, or there may be young children sharing rooms with a dying patient; both young and old are likely to suffer from this experience. There has been far too much generalization in the discussions about the proper place to die, each death is an individual experience and the doctor needs to assess the facilities for each patient. This will inevitably involve consultation between the hospital doctor, the general practitioner, the district nurse, the social worker, relatives, and friends.

Whatever the decision, it may be necessary to change it later, depending on the ensuing circumstances, and either admit the patient to hospital or discharge him home. The facilities available through the social services for the provision of essential requirements at home have greatly eased some of the problems of home-care.

A correct attitude to death is perhaps more easily achieved in a special home, where those around the patient are used to the problems of the dying and the patient in the next bed is in the same state. It is to be expected that there will develop an atmosphere of compassion, concern, dignity, and even of interest in one another and in everyday things going on around; that friendships will spring up between patients and that they will share in sorrow, in distress, in joy, in hope. Dying at home or in the busy hospital ward produces quite different circumstances. At home there is concern, upset at seeing the distress in the faces of relatives and friends; quietness there may be but perhaps also boredom, and the patient may be alone for periods of time during the day. In the hospital ward of a busy clinical unit there is the extreme of noise and bustle, the agony of being moved to the dreaded bed near the door, or the side-ward, the possibility that people are too busily concerned with the care of the living to spare more than an occasional glance at those who no longer need such care. It is difficult sometimes for the doctor to assume the right approach to an individual patient, to show interest in his voice, his looks, his examination. Frequently he has made up his mind that nothing more can be done and it is not easy to disguise this; he may end up by giving the patient the impression that he is too busy, bored, or has better and more important things to do. We are all guilty of this and it is hard not to be otherwise.

Doctors must also recognize that the patient sometimes does not want to be disturbed or talked to; there are times in life when we all feel a need for solitude – 'alone with our thoughts' – these will occur also at the time of death. There are also times when the patient needs to cry without being consoled or discouraged. There are times when he wants to see people and have them by him but silent, times he may not wish to eat and nothing will be lost if he does not. The doctor needs to respect these times. Usually in his clinical practice he is more concerned with encouraging his patient or even mildly bullying him or urging him on to progress in spite of his discomfort; in terminal illness there must be an entirely different approach dictated not by the doctor but by the patient. Finally, every doctor must realize the uselessness of investigations which do not improve the patient's well-being and may even cause him concern or discomfort.

It is perhaps pertinent for the doctor in assessing his attitude to the terminal care of the cancer patient to consider his own demise, for:

It is a thing that everyone suffers, even persons of the lowest resolution, of the meanest virtue, of no breeding, of no discourse. Take away but the pomp of death, the disguises and solemn bugbears, the tinsel and the actings by candle-light, and the proper and fantastic ceremonies, the minstrels and the noise makers, the women and the weepers, the swoonings and the shriekings, the nurses and the physicians, the dark room and the ministers, the kindred and the watchers and then to die is easy, ready and quitted from its troublesome circumstances. It is the same harmless thing that a poor shepherd suffered yesterday, or a maid-servant today; and at the same time in which you die, in that very night a thousand creatures die with you, some wise men, and many fools; and the wisdom of the first will not quit him, and the folly of the latter does not make him unable to die.

(Bishop Jeremy Taylor (1613–67), *Holy Dying*)

Death

Death can arouse practically every possible emotion: sorrow, despair, pain, grief, regret, anger, dislike, fear, anxiety, apprehension, terror, affection, love, benevolence, respect, surprise, curiosity, and even admiration. But perhaps behind all these emotions there is one that occupies a paramount place, and that is fear.

> Men fear death as children fear to go in the dark, and as that natural fear in children is increased with tales, so is the other.
> (Francis Bacon (1561–1626), *Of Death*)

Fear of death is a basic emotion which is experienced by all and the doctor will share in this fear, which may be influenced to a degree by his own knowledge. If, for example, he is accustomed to dealing with a lesion carrying a poor prognosis and associated pain and suffering, he may consider death as a happy release from distress.

There is an attitude of the doctor's mind that demands special examination and which is probably more prevalent than is at first thought, the doctor's belief that death has occurred because he has failed. Trained throughout his life to heal, to alleviate pain and suffering, to attempt to cure, it is inevitable that he should consider anything less than these as failure. Our whole approach to malignant disease is based on an assessment of 'cure' or survival; comparisons are made of differing techniques of treatment or operation and are compared with the results of other workers. Death from other causes, intercurrent diseases, or accidents, are counted against us and we view them as if they were deliberately inserted to reduce our results. It is possible that unconsciously this feeling of failure may result in the clinician losing some interest in his patient. This may arise in several ways; he may feel embarrassed by the patient's continuing faith and hope that a cure will be obtained, or he may develop a desire to blot from his mind all thoughts of an unpleasant failure. Acceptance of death is as necessary in the doctor's as it is in the patient's mind.

It must be appreciated that death in malignant disease is usually not an abrupt occurrence but progresses over a period of time until there comes a point of 'no return' which may last for several days before the end. A prevailing clinical attitude is that 'while there is life there is hope'. Associated with this is the feeling prevalent among radiotherapists that once a course of treatment has been planned it should be proceeded with as long as the patient is alive; the result is that sometimes a patient who is steadily deteriorating may be treated even on the day of his death. In defence of this we must point out that it is not always easy to know when a patient is going to die; but a more critical approach must be taken if the patient is to be spared un-necessary disturbance.

A doctor's attitude may be influenced by his beliefs; this effectively comes down to whether he believes death to be episodal or catastrophic, whether it is merely a point in the whole organization of existence, or the fatal end. Whatever his belief, he must be careful not to antagonize the beliefs of his patient if they are sustaining him at this time.

The doctor with his desire to preserve life must accept that the patient may well know the seriousness of his condition and may not wish to go on when such life is only obtained at a premium and may produce distress and discomfort. He will not wish the doctor to miss any opportunity of cure, but he may well want to avoid unnecessary discomfort. Death may indeed by a happy release from long suffering and despair. We must recognize that patients may dread not so much the death as the process of dying and the thought that they may be kept alive lingering in fear without release. This has been noted by many writers, thus:

> Vital spark of heav'nly flame!
> Quit, oh quit this mortal frame:
> Trembling, hoping, ling'ring, flying,
> Oh the pain, the bliss of dying.
>
> (Alexander Pope (1688–1744),
> *The Dying Christian to his Soul*)

Post-mortem examinations are an essential source of medical knowledge, and the attitudes about these vary from hospital to hospital. In some it is almost accepted as a routine; in others it is only carried out if the relatives are specifically consulted, or if there is a reason why the cause of death cannot be accurately determined. If relatives are approached and there appears to be no logical reason for such an examination, it is inevitable that there will be reluctance about interfering with the body. This whole question requires very careful handling; there must be respect for the dead and for the relatives, and a balance must be struck between this and the search for knowledge which may help future patients.

PREPAREDNESS
It prudently behoves all men to prepare for the time of death and to make adequate preparation; failure to do so results in insecurity for those left behind. Mundane matters such as the disposal of property may need to be decided by Court Order with all the upset, distress, and uncertainty associated with such procedures. Wives and families, though provided for, need to await formal recognition of their rights before they can obtain sufficient of their own to provide for their everyday needs. Financial embarrassment may result for the surviving spouse at a time when she is least able to cope. Making a will is a normal procedure and responsibility for each and every one of us; more so for a man who has the obligations of a wife and family. Unfortunately there is reluctance and almost a feeling of superstition against such a preparation. In a technological age when accidents abound, when sudden death is not uncommmon, it would appear a necessity.

It is not always easy to advise a patient at a time when he knows or suspects that he is seriously ill. Making a will should be a procedure carried out calmly in normal health, not 'hurriedly and worriedly' in sickness. It would be desirable if some national attempt was made to persuade people to set their affairs in order, based purely on a rational response to the need. It is an attitude of mind that could usefully be encouraged. In any case the patient should be persuaded to do so as a matter of routine when he is admitted to hospital.

Euthanasia

Literally, euthanasia means a good death (Greek: *eu* – well, *thanatos* – death), but it has become associated with the deliberate putting to death of a person, especially of patients with incurable disease. In primitive races there were obvious reasons for killing the old; migrant tribes who depended on travelling for food would be held up by the old and infirm, tribes pursued by enemies would be hindered in their escape, so frequently the old were left behind with the minimum of necessities. This was particularly seen in certain North American Indian tribes, the Wailakki, Poncas, Omahas, and so on.

However, some tribes made deliberate efforts to spare the infirm any further privations or abuse from enemies and deliberately killed them; for example, the Tupis in Brazil, the Tobas in Paraguay, and certain natives of Australia. The victims were killed by burying alive, by jumping or being thrown off a cliff, strangulation, or poison. In many cases death was with the approval of the victim; it was an accepted tribal practice and could be demanded by the aged or infirm as a right. Improvements in social status and in community security have now eliminated these necessities. In more recent years, however, there has been a demand to kill those with incurable diseases who request it, and the Voluntary Euthanasia Society was founded in 1935 with the idea of promoting legislation for voluntary death. Three Bills have been presented unsuccessfully to Parliament, in 1936, 1950, and 1969.

It has been claimed that euthanasia is justified because the decision to demand this to be carried out when necessary has been made by the patient not at a time of stress caused by illness, or the proximity of death, or pain, but well beforehand when he was fit and could make a rational decision.

There are many arguments against euthanasia; briefly these are:

(a)   It would be difficult to adopt any form of legislation without leaving open the possibility of abuse by the relatives, or even the doctor, or by the patient who has either no desire for life (legalized suicide), or believes himself to be a burden to his relatives or friends, or those whom he loves.

(b)   Killing is antipathetic to man's beliefs; it is against all ideas of human dignity, is socially and morally wrong, is opposed to the high level of responsibility demanded of humans, and is antagonistic to the basic human feeling of compassion and forgiveness. Hence, many communities have already abolished the death penalty. It is unfortunate that man, whilst expressing such high ideals, can at the same time excuse the futile waste of life that occurs in war and in such aggressive opposition that allows the killing of defenceless and innocent individuals by using force to achieve political ends.

(c)   It is against the teaching and practice of doctors:

I will use treatment to help the sick according to my

ability and judgement, but never with a view to injury or wrong doing. Neither will I administer a poison to anybody when asked to do so, nor will I suggest such a course (Hippocratic Oath).

It has been suggested that not only must the doctor decide that the condition is incurable but also that death should come by his hand; he thus becomes judge and executioner. On what medical criteria can it be justified? On suffering and pain? But usually these can be relieved. On the patient's desire for death? But who is he to anticipate nature? For economic reasons, because he is a drain on the community? But the community exists to help those who are afflicted and indeed makes the necessary economic arrangements for this. Certainly it would be necessary to have several medical opinions; doctors, as others, are liable to bias, mistaken thinking, and eccentricities, and are influenced by their own attitudes or even by unsound judgement. But even if the doctor makes the decision, it cannot be by him that death is brought about; this is totally against all the ethics of medical practice.

(d) The need for euthanasia was reputedly based on terminal suffering, but modern analgesics and the improved and enlightened approach to terminal care have to a great extent removed the necessity. Many patients dying of malignant disease live a full, interesting, and painless life right up to the end.

(e) Killing is against many religious beliefs; for example, the Judaeo-Christian sixth commandment is 'Thou shalt not kill'. Similar admonitions are made in other faiths and other communities. Euthanasia is abhorrent to the thinking of many doctors and to most other people, but perhaps the most important thing is that there is no real need for it. What is required is a more rational approach to death, a realization of the needs of the dying person, practical application of medical measures to relieve pain and suffering, maintenance of the individual's dignity, and attempts at removing the fear, not so much the fear of death itself but that of dying. The doctor can help by being willing to talk about death and helping to prepare the patient in body, mind, and spirit.

8

Attitudes to Communication – Secrecy

Communication

A considerable volume of literature has been written about what should be told to the patient. I have no desire to add materially to this but would like merely to point out various facets which may affect the doctor's attitude to his patient. It is important to realize two things; firstly, that both doctor and patient are individuals, and, secondly, that the responsibility of the doctor is to care for his patient. Now, care means not only that the best is done to help the patient materially and physically in his illness but also that nothing is done to upset or worry him.

We have been told at length about the patient's rights, especially his right to know the full nature of his disease and the prognosis, but it must be pointed out that it is seldom the patient or his relatives who demand these rights but rather that others demand them for him. Many of these people do it with the best intent, but unfortunately more in the way of criticism than of thought for the person who is ill. Lord Justice Edmund Davies ('The Patient's Right to Know the Truth', *Proceedings of the Royal Society of Medicine*, vol. 66, 1973) considered the patient's right to know the truth, and the duty of the doctor to tell him, and concluded that 'in general no such legal duty exists'. To quote further:

> What the law requires is no more (and no less) than reasonable care and skill in the treatment of each particular patient. Beyond that, it refuses to generalize, and this for what we regard as good reasons. For just as the medicine a doctor prescribes and the surgeon advises will vary with each patient so will the extent to which the doctor lifts the veil. At the threshold there arises the question: What patient and what truth? To tell the truth to some may be brutal, despite their entreaties; to withold it from others may be a massive mistake. In deciding what is the proper course in the particular case lies the art of medicine.

Obviously the decision whether or not to tell the patient is a medical responsibility and invariably the doctor is the best person to advise. The doctor will justifiably demand that if the patient is to be told it will be communicated in a way which produces as little harm as possible to both patient and relatives. We must as far as possible do no harm.

In arriving at his decision of what to tell, the doctor will balance the opposing effects of knowledge of the truth and of ignorance, based upon his own knowledge of the disease, its prognosis, the possible effects on the patient, and of the patient's background, mental state, and so on. It is preposterous to think that he may be deliberately hiding the truth and that this could be to the patient's detriment. Harm can be caused by telling the truth and equally harm may result from withholding it.

The problems of telling are resolved by a series of questions; Should the patient be told? Who should tell him? What should be told? When should he be told? Where should he be told? Who else should be told? It is impossible to deal adequately with these questions separately; they are of course interrelated, and the answer to one question affects the others. However, we shall try very briefly to point out some possible answers.

SHOULD THE PATIENT BE TOLD?

The answer is 'yes' if at all possible and if the doctor is sure that the patient can appreciate the answers and that these will do him no harm. Religious beliefs are involved: the practising Christian is prepared for death, which in a way holds few fears for him, and these are minimal if, as a result of his religious beliefs, he also believes in a life after death and even more so if already he has lived a full and useful life. The doctor's information only confirms what he already knows. The patient who is ill and has been admitted to hospital and who is slowly deteriorating must be aware of his failing health, more so if he has received such specialist treatment as radiotherapy. But he may not wish to discuss his approaching death and indeed he may create a fantasy that all is well and that he will recover. He may 'opt out' and completely close his mind to such problems. In these circumstances, telling him may not be the best thing; indeed with some patients there is resistance to being told and to understanding.

WHO SHOULD TELL?

Usually the expert's opinion is best, the doctor who has made the diagnosis or the family doctor who has known the patient for many years; either will accept it as a duty or responsibility. Support will come from clergy, social workers, nurses, relations, and friends.

WHAT SHOULD BE TOLD?

The patient should be told in simple unequivocal language; it is, I believe, better to say a few simple words sympathetically but clearly than to try to cover up or circumnavigate. The patient in his state of anxiety and stress is avid for factual information; it is very easy to give the wrong impression and to leave him in a state of doubt. It is unecessary perhaps to state that the information must be given quietly and kindly; brutal facts can cause irreparable hurt and the resultant embarrassment breaks down the rapport between doctor and patient which will be essential in the ensuing months. The patient may then request to be left alone or may have questions to ask and the doctor must be prepared for either alternative.

WHEN SHOULD HE BE TOLD?

It is important that information is given at the right time if at all possible, and here we must take into account popular belief that cancer is a hopeless, fatal disease. Over-optimism may arouse doubts; why if I have a simple disease should I have such a large operation or a protracted course of treatment and then come regularly for follow-up examination after? It is important to obtain a due sense of balance. It may be preferable to tell the patient that he has a serious condition, that there is every hope that he will be cured if he undergoes treatment, and that the doctor will keep a careful eye on him afterwards. It is hoped that as a result the patient will appreciate the need for co-operation and that he will be anxious to help. Should his condition deteriorate he will be told more: that the disease is still not under control, that further treatment is needed; and eventually he will be told that the condition is fatal. By this time he will have become gradually adjusted to this knowledge. Important then to tell at the right time, not too early to destroy hope, nor too late so that suspicions are aroused and faith and co-operation negated.

WHERE?
Without doubt he should be told in privacy; it cannot be done in a busy out-patient department or ward. If at all possible the patient should be taken into a side ward or a separate room, made comfortable, and told quietly, without embarrassment or fuss.

WHO ELSE?
Whether or not we decide to tell the patient, a close or responsible relative should be informed of the full details. The general practitioner usually knows the most responsible relative. It may be desirable that a spouse is not told if he is elderly, ill, or emotional. But delay or hiding the truth may be undesirable; preparedness for a loved one's death is usually preferable to immediate shock. Discussion will reveal whether it is a good thing for husband and wife, one of whom has cancer, to talk it over together. A man and wife married for many years are used to discussing things together whether they are good things or bad, and to talk together at the time of worry about one's illness may help each of them to face the ultimate moment of separation and enable the survivor to carry helpful memories after the event. There may be some consolation for them to know that they both have discussed the future and even planned it together. In these days children are more aware of death than we sometimes give them credit for. Considerable trauma may be caused if a parent is abruptly removed from them; they should be prepared for the death, if possible, and in this way also they may bring affection and comfort to the dying parent. It is difficult to be dogmatic, but I believe that even young children can be told, though the way in which they are told depends on the individual child and his age. The doctor may be the best person to tell them, or a responsible relative or the surviving parent. However much the doctor may regret or even dislike telling, it is his responsibility if requested to do so by the relatives. Children can be unbelievably helpful when a difficult task has to be done, and sometimes I have been grateful to the child for his willingness to help me to convey a very difficult message. It is important that the child feels that he is being brought into the confidence of the grown-ups rather than that he is ignored or rejected.

Telling the patient and his relatives is by no means the simple task that some would have us believe, there are no clear rules and every patient must be treated as an individual; that at least is his right. Each patient, each relative, indeed each doctor, is an individual; the possible permutations of the attitudes of approach are infinite. Those who try to generalize reveal only their relative inexperience of the problems. Whatever we do must be to the advantage firstly of the patient and secondly of the relatives, but it must in no way do harm.

Secrecy

There is always an aura of mystery to the conclaves of medical men. One may wonder whether the secrecy with which the fraternity surrounds its gathering is designed to keep the layman from discovering how much it knows or how much it doesn't know. Either knowledge would be unnerving to that immemorial guinea pig who submits himself to the abracadabra of chemicals, scalpels and incantations under the delusion he is being cured rather than explored.

(Ben Hecht (1893–1964), *Miracle of fifteen murders*)

This quotation aptly summarizes the feeling of some lay people to the doctor's secrecy. Frequently this stems from a desire to protect the patient from knowledge which may cause him harm, distress, or unhappiness. Indeed it may be that the doctor's special knowledge leads him to assume a vague approach so that the patient seeks no further information. We must also admit that frequently we do not know and that instead of confessing this we attempt to keep quiet. The doctor has the advantage that frequently he can make an intelligent guess whereas the patient is only confused. If the doctor is going to maintain a policy of secrecy to patient and relatives he must make sure that it is interpreted correctly and that he recognizes the possible effects on a family who are not informed of the possible outcome of the disease.

Professionally we have maintained a policy of secrecy to cancer for many years, but this is now being broken down by attempts to instruct the general public. It is hoped that research and medical education will help us to take a more realistic approach to the giving of such information.

9

Others Concerned with Cancer

We must remember the many others who are concerned with patient care – these include scientists, nurses, social workers, radiographers, receptionists, porters, ward orderlies, domestic workers, secretaries, clerks, engineers, ambulance drivers, and so on. We can conveniently divide these into two groups; those who come into direct contact with the patient and those who do not, and it is the first group which concerns us. The approach to the attitudes of these people is very like that previously discussed when we related them to the doctor; there is, therefore, no need to reiterate them.

Whilst we may spend time instructing many people in their approach to the patient, we may forget some who have a direct relationship which is not at first obvious. Patients very often feel ill at ease with doctors, nurses, and ancillary medical workers whom they presume to have an almost mystical knowledge: as a result they are frequently diffident about asking questions. However, they may approach others who may appear to be somewhat nearer to them; thus, the ward orderly or domestic worker as she cleans the ward may be taken into the patient's confidence and be questioned. Porters may be asked about the illness as they push patients along hospital corridors. Questions may be naïvely phrased – thus, 'It is true that I have cancer, isn't it?', may lead the porter or other to think that the patient has been told and he will assent, but the patient may have a benign lesion and in his desire to avoid discussion the porter's assent may lead the patient to be wrongly informed. We need to be careful of trick questions aimed at someone who does not know.

The attitude of these other workers cannot and should not be ignored; frequently they have strong feelings about the patients and wish to do hospital work because of this. It is important to accept that all these workers are part of the caring team. We must therefore not only accept them but give them some understanding of the work that is being done in the hospital. We must help them to form a positive attitude to malignant disease; too often they have little or no knowledge and adopt the popular view that this is a hopeless disease. As a result they prefer not to talk to cancer patients or, if they do, show only too plainly what they think. Specially designed hospitals treating cancer patients, wards devoted to cancer patients, and terminal homes manage to instill into their staff the need for care in talking to the patients. One can only stress the importance of the 'team work'; this is obvious in a small hospital, especially one devoted to cancer, but becomes a little lost in the large and very large hospital. The ward sister is in a unique position to give some elementary information and to back this up with informal discussions. She too will help to convince these workers of the important role they have to play. Unfortunately only too frequently many of us take their work for granted. Opportunities should be given for discussion and it would help to give suitable instruction to porters, domestic staff, and other workers.

Conclusion

Our studies have demonstrated two important aspects of medical attitudes, the *inherent factor* and the *environmental factor* represented to a large extent respectively by 'fear' and 'experience'. Incomplete knowledge limits the full appreciation of the disease and sullies the mental attitude, a state which can only be remedied by seeking further knowledge. This in turn produces the realization that something can be done for this disease. We have adequate information that the results of treatment can be improved as a result of investigation and research, and also that the discovery of further aetiological factors may help us to devise methods of preventing at least some of the cancers.

There is thus little support for the defeatist attitude adopted by some doctors who have grouped all malignant disease under the one common heading of 'cancer' and have applied the worst possible prognosis to the whole group. For, like 'infection', 'cancer' is a generic term applied to a mixed group of diseases where the outcome varies tremendously. We must adopt the right attitude to the right malignant disease. Some patients are cured with little or no permanent effect and that disease should be viewed with more realistic optimism; a more pessimistic approach continues to be necessary for some other malignancies but it should be tempered with the knowledge that what can be done for some cancers may, with further research, become possible for even the worst.

There can be little doubt that the future attack on malignant diseases will depend to a great extent on the attitude of the individual doctor whose responsibility is the cure of the individual patient.

10

The Patient

As personal experience of malignant diseases grows, it becomes more usual to develop an attitude more aligned to the disease than to the individual. The doctor and nurse have invariably seen many such patients and have a very good idea of the possible outcome of treatment. They may be forgiven, therefore, for not appreciating to the full the individual patient's concern. This attitude perhaps develops because of familiarity with the disease, as a means of shielding the patient, or merely because of sheer overwork with large numbers of patients. Inevitably each new patient is in danger of being accepted as 'another one'. We, as doctors, may be criticized for this approach, but it fits the management of the individual case – a routine adopted by the doctor, nurse, department, or ward in which it is possible to give maximal patient care without missing anything out or being involved. In a way the patient responds favourably to this stereotyped care because he then believes that it is something routine, that the staff are familiar and confident, and that there is a pattern which he can follow. Indeed, our modern society accepts such conformity.

We must now examine the reactions of the patient to all the possible outcomes of cancer – the fear that it may develop, the presence of symptoms leading to suspicion, to detection and investigation, to probable, possible, and definite diagnosis, to operation or treatment, to aftercare, rehabilitation, terminal illness, and approaching death. These must be looked at in two ways which are not entirely separate, as the herd instinct and as the individual attitude. We shall find many variations in the possible responses, and it will be necessary to generalize at times. We must accept that no one wants this disease, that the vast majority have very little knowledge of it, that there are many varying responses in the cancer patient depending on the symptoms, the response to treatment, and the outcome, and also that inevitably the patient's attitude is biased.

Cancerphobia

Worry will, of course, play an important role in the response of the patient who has cancer, but some patients may fear the possibility of developing it to such an extent that it warrants the term 'phobia'.

It is normal to experience some anxiety about the possibility of developing a cancer, and this is frequently 'triggered off' by a recent event, a relative or friend diagnosed as having cancer, information through one of the media, or unusual personal symptoms. This normal anxiety may last a few days and may even precipitate a visit to the doctor but soon settles – it is merely one of the worries associated with living in modern society. In some patients, however, no such causal factor exists and the anxiety may assume major importance to the extent that the patient spends a considerable time worrying about it.

Patients with cancerphobia have a sincere problem; they are convinced that they have malignant disease but are unable to convince those who they think could and should give treatment. Attempts at reassurance frequently do not work and they seek other medical opinions. At times their fear is general – 'I am sure I have a cancer somewhere' – this may be associated with a general anxiety state or being physically run-down. The implication is that only a cancer could produce such a condition. Others have a definite fear of a cancer at a certain site. The latter often has an exciting cause, for example a relative – often the mother – who had cancer at some time in her life and the patient is convinced that she, too, will suffer in the same way. Alternatively he may have a definite long-standing disease which has been diagnosed but which does not clear as rapidly as he would wish – 'so obviously there is something more'. This is found with many chronic diseases, such as cystitis or bronchitis, and sufferers develop a mental attitude which suspects that the doctor is deceiving them by making a benign diagnosis to cover up the underlying fatal one.

Some of these patients may be suffering from genuine psychiatric problems, others may merely be following the whims of fashion. The phobics may thus be genuinely worried or merely seeking popularity or sympathy, but they must never be ignored and need to be examined and reassured.

Diagnosis

The patient with symptoms is anxious to have them diagnosed and treatment started – or, at least, one would imagine this to be the case. But, in many cases of malignant disease, there is a long clinical history, sometimes of months, even years, in patients who are reluctant to have an examination.

Malcolm Donaldson dedicated his book *The Cancer Riddle* (1933) to 'thousands of patients in the past who have died due to Fear and Ignorance of the disease, which has prevented them from seeking medical advice at a time when, in many cases, the disease would have been curable'.

Delay may occur because the patient is occupied, is afraid, ignorant, ascetic, or credulous. Many people have lives crowded with appointments, meetings, and committees; housewives often work to supplement the family finances, leisure time is filled with either active sports or passive radio and television, there is little time to think and none for meeting the unexpected. It may be that this is merely an excuse, but for many the illness is ill-timed, they will come later 'after haymaking' or 'harvest' or 'ploughing' and so on. Others may have conflicting interests; we all prefer to do the interesting rather than the more exacting or worrying. Many simply fear the unknown; they dread the possible outcome of their symptoms, their possible embarrassment or inadequacy to meet the situation, or even the unfamiliarity of approaching the doctor. Some hope that by their delaying the symptoms will go away, or plead that haste is unseemly; this may be no more than an escapist attitude. They may know no better and be unaware that they should seek advice; alternatively they may actively resist. The ascetic may deny the failings of the body or may believe that he can overcome the disease, ignore it, or wish it away. The credulous may oppose medical aid because of his religious or other beliefs or because he has no faith in doctors. Inaccurate knowledge in the wiseacre may lead him to believe that nothing can be done.

Delay and procrastination are elementary human failings, but cancer is an acute disease and delay can mean dissemination with a consequent poor prognosis.

Verification

The patient attends the doctor and hospital and the presence of malignant disease is confirmed. Many patients respond with profound shock and bewilderment, no tenseness, no concern, no crying or despair, just a stunned numbness. It may be some time before this wears off: in some patients it may take minutes, in others hours or even days, occasionally never. I believe that this is not a time for the doctor to persist in or to elaborate his explanations: further exposition is not appreciated or is incompletely so and leads to even further bewilderment. There is a possibility that as a result the patient may conceive incorrect information which it is difficult to correct, or indeed may never be corrected, and may jeopardize the relationship between him and his doctor.

The next move comes from the patient who will ask questions when he is ready; these must be answered simply, straightforwardly, and correctly, without any attempt at concealment of facts. Whatever the intelligence of the patient his shocked condition demands that questions are answered in simple language. Each point must be carefully put and appreciated before proceeding to the next.

This period of numbness and incomplete realization of the facts may indeed last for some time if the patient is fully occupied and other things are happening; for example, a patient will proceed through a course of radiotherapy almost as an automaton, doing what he is told, not asking questions, quiet, withdrawn, and obviously worried. Attempts to communicate with him at this time may result in failure, as he is not receptive. Completion of the treatment brings with it a change from what has been an acceptable routine and poses new problems. These are associated with the future and the answers will incite further questions, hopes, and fears and perhaps a realization of the full nature of the illness. It is at this time that a sympathetic explanation of the facts becomes essential. Subsequent adjustment to the idea of having a cancer occurs in the majority of people.

Depression to some degree and at some time is a natural instinct; it may occur at the time of diagnosis or may be associated with some family event such as an anniversary or birthday. It may also occur when treatment appears to be unsuccessful, when further therapy has to be given, as a result of toxic products produced during radiation, and, inevitably, in the terminal stage of the disease. It is a natural response to disappointment, loss, or worry; however, it may escalate to such a stage that the patient attempts suicide. Physical illnesses account for up to thirty per cent of cases of depression, and cancer is an important contributing cause. Suicide for various reasons has increased in most countries; many attempts are somewhat half-hearted, but the cancer patient who has reached a sufficiently depressed state to wish death is determined, he has a strong desire forced upon him by the apparent inevitability of the disease. Even if he is subsequently cured of his cancer, his suicidal tendency may remain; he is not convinced that his treatment was successful, and psychiatric help may be necessary.

Readjustment to normal life after a diagnosis of cancer has been made comes slowly, indeed it only comes after there is overwhelming evidence of the effectiveness of the treatment. At this time support has to be given by many people: the patient's immediate relatives, friends, close acquaintances, clergy, nurses, radiographers, medical social workers, and doctors. Seldom does he have the opportunity of receiving support from members of the community who have been cured. Organizations are formed to help many patients, such as those who have had colostomies, laryngectomies, amputations, or who are diabetics or spastics, and the members obtain considerable moral support from seeing the way in which others have coped with their illness or disability. But cancer is an anonymous disease and the result is that there are no groups of successfully treated patients able to give support to those who have recently been diagnosed; indeed many of those cured, well, and living normal lives, are unaware of the true nature of their original illness.

Blame

Man is persuaded that to every effect there is a cause, so if cancer develops usually someone, or more usually something, must be blamed and these include habits, pastimes, previous illnesses, or injuries. The family doctor is at times accused of missing symptoms or of delaying the consultant, of procrastination, or of inadequate or inappropriate treatment. Occasionally the family may be blamed, frequently God. Much of this is a search for a scapegoat. The patient may decide that it is a result of his own wrongdoing – at times of stress it is sometimes fantastic to find what normal circumstances can assume bizarre characteristics; this applies particularly to personal morals and habits.

Communication

I have touched briefly on the problems of communication but they are considerable. The specialist frequently finds difficulty in making it clear to his patient, and no wonder; he is trying to express what he has accumulated in many years of specialized work in a simple way to a distressed patient, in a few brief minutes. A man who is accustomed to lecturing, writing, and discussing at a professional level with colleagues often finds it difficult to write or talk at *Reader's Digest* level, and fails because often even that level is too high for his patient. Specialists in any discipline, profession, or trade find the same problems.

A natural desire to shield may lead to the doctor giving the wrong information. The patient inevitably wants to communicate and to know because everything is strange, bewildering, frightening. Communication between doctor and patient need not be oral or written but may be by means of a less defined sense, a 'feeling', or 'atmosphere' based, perhaps, on faith or confidence. I am reminded of the old farmer who opened his letter in front of the postman, looked at it and smiled contentedly; questioned about the blank pages he replied that he could neither read or write and the sender, his brother, was similarly limited but they *communicated*.

The Doctor

Relationships between doctor and patient are subject to change over the years and with the type of medicine practised, whether nationalized, private, insurance, and so on. The relationships may also vary with the disease present, and this can be particularly true of cancer. A kind of love-hate relationship exists alternating between the reverenced healer and the quack or mountebank – with this disease the doctor is not credited with previous successes because these are unknown. The relationship is therefore on a somewhat shaky, artificial basis. Regrettably sometimes there is almost a pantomime, the doctor attempting to believe the patient doesn't know the diagnosis, the patient fearing to establish the true facts, hence creating a charade of relationships. Again this may be instigated by fear and ignorance on the patient's side and compassion and disguise on the doctor's.

Pessimism may cause the patient to reject the treatment; we are all familiar with the patient who 'gives up' and refuses to co-operate even though the prognosis is good. In these cases persuasion may need to be augmented by command or force which may be interpreted as aggression. It is important that the patient is not given the impression that he is rejected because he has a hopeless prognosis. An *inability* to do more by the doctor may occasionally be interpreted as *unwillingness* to do more. Being beyond help is a not uncommon feeling among patients and must be countered if possible, but attempts to do this may produce alternating feelings of co-operation and a need for attention and resentment or even aggression towards the doctor. It is an expression of insecurity and of fear. The patient frequently recognizes this and, after an outburst of difficult relationships with his doctor, is apologetic and filled with remorse. All those dealing with patients need to be aware of these problems and must try to avoid provocation. Jeremy Taylor exhorted patients to obey their physicians and 'not to be ungently and uneasy to the ministers and nurses that attend us, but to take their diligent and kind offices as sweetly as we can and to bear their indiscretions or unhandsome accidents contentedly and without disquietness within or evil language or angry words without'. Good advice, perhaps, but perhaps not applicable to modern society.

Anger may result from the hopelessness of the condition, from resentment that 'it has happened to me', from distress at the cutting short of a career or of proposals for the future, or from fear or worry about family, and other factors. This anger may be directed towards the doctor for his failure to cure. There is a growing belief that the doctor should know, should cure, and that if he does not he is failing in his duty. This is perhaps a continuation of ancient beliefs where the doctor was punished for not curing.

After-care and Rehabilitation

The idea that cancer is not curable accounts perhaps for the patient's reluctance to assume a normal existence again, and this belief is often supported by his relatives. Thus, the cured patient may need some persuasion to resume his previous occupation or a lighter one; to take a positive rather than a negative approach. Many patients do return to normal and do so in spite of permanent complications, prostheses, or disabilities. The doctor needs to encourage this return whenever possible; self-respect is best achieved if a man feels that he is pulling his weight in the house and is a breadwinner. A positive approach to rehabilitation can be achieved more easily if there is social and economic security, and the social services therefore have much to offer. Again, persuasion may be needed to accept 'charity' when this is required.

Considerable reassurance can be given to the patient about the outcome of treatment before his operation or therapy. We can again consider the patient who notices a lump in the breast; worried, she attends her doctor and is referred to hospital. She may be told she is to be admitted, then she will have an operation to biopsy the growth and depending on what is found she may wake up from the anaesthetic with only a small incision or having had the breast removed. The indecision naturally leads her to be worried. Alternatively, drill biopsy taken in out-patients can provide a paraffin section for definite histological diagnosis and a result is obtained within twenty-four hours. If it is a cancer the patient is prepared for an operation, told what this will entail, and is introduced to the fitting of an artificial breast. This, then, is a planned operation rather than 'we shall see what we find'. Now removal of the breast may have quite a devastating effect on some patients; femininity is associated with this organ, body-shape is an essential female attribute to be proud of, removal signifies rejection by husband, family, and society – an exaggerated response maybe, but certainly present. A convincing breast prosthesis is essential to the patient's subsequent peace of mind. The breast has weight, it moves with body movement, swinging on the chest muscles, it has shape usually symmetrical with the opposite side. Cotton wool stuffed into a brassière lacks weight, does not move with body movements and will slip; sorbo rubber is little better, inflated balloons lack weight and may puncture, glycerol in a shaped bag has weight but also sets up a wave motion. New prostheses made up of small plastic spheres are very good substitutes and give the patient confidence. The prosthesis should be fitted with a normal dress brassière, feminine, nicely shaped and not the usual surgical type, which is somewhat heavy, rough, strengthened, and far from a feminine piece of dress. Time taken to fit an artificial breast is important.

A similar story can be made for all other prostheses – the important thing to remember is individual fitting, adequate preparation to accept it, and perseverance by the patient.

Terminal Care

It is important to retain the patient's dignity and individuality at the time of death. Many people fear the act of dying far more than they do the actual death.

There is reluctance to leave the familiar and those we know, fear maybe of the actual process of dying. Will I manage? Is it degrading? Is there pain? Generally the older the patient the more he accepts it, especially if the spouse is already dead. Our attitudes to death are dictated by our knowledge, experience, reading, upbringing, and not least of all by our religious beliefs. The Christian looks for a life beyond, other faiths assume that this world is hell and that life only begins after death, paradise is reserved for a particular community . . . there are numerous approaches, but to many death is a termination. The imaginative Victorian approach to death was suitable to a more fanciful age; this modern technical age concerned as it is with fact sees little beyond the grave. Thus religious beliefs may affect the prevailing attitude; peace of mind and preparedness may bring about a quiet resignation. Pain, as we have already seen, can be controlled in the majority of patients although this knowledge is lacking in many lay people, even in some doctors and nurses. It is an achievement to keep the patient alive enjoying life as much as he can, free from pain, secure among friends until this time comes; he should be living fully, conscious that he is not alone. We are fortunate that often death in cancer is not a sudden process but takes place over a period of some days during which there is a gradual sinking, an insensible acceptance. Some dying patients attempt to draw a curtain between them and their friends and associates, but such separation can be detrimental to them, to the relatives, and to the health care team.

This generation is fully conversant with dying, with hunger, want, and war; the consequent cheapening of human life induces an acceptance of unnatural suffering and death. But there is fear of dying, of pain, of suffering, and of lingering on, of life being prolonged, hence the plea – 'when the time comes let my passing be smooth, that I may not linger in pain with no hope, a burden on those I love'.

Conclusion

The points that we have mentioned are varied and complex and there are many combinations and permutations that shape the attitude of the patient to the knowledge that he has malignant disease. Just as each patient is an individual, so his approach will be characteristic, and attitudes may change depending on circumstances; there is no standard patient and we must not generalize.

11

Current Attitudes of the Relatives

The relatives' immediate reaction to the diagnosis is that the patient will suffer and that death is inevitable; this is soon followed by questions about their own future. The reactions will, of course, depend on the closeness of the relationship, the particular nature of the disease, the age of the patient, and will be conditioned by how much the relative and patient are told.

Giving information to a relative is not always easy; invariably it is done at visiting time when the doctor is busy and has other relatives or patients to see, and, more often than not, it is given by a junior doctor. There is naturally some stress when a relative is told at the beginning of visiting time and then has to 'put on a brave face' to see the patient and try to keep up a pretence. If possible, such discussions should be left until the end of visiting; a cup of tea always helps and the relative should have a few minutes alone to readjust before going off. When it can be managed a small private room should be available for this interview. Unfortunately, interviews with relatives are not a routine; we get complaints from relatives that they were never told, which brings the response that they never asked. Now both are in a way logical arguments, perhaps because both sides have attempted to avoid the responsibility. The relatives need to know, but some do not ask because they are afraid to disturb busy doctors or nurses – they have been informed for years how busy these people are – some are afraid to know the true answer, some do not want to know, some are nervous about asking, thinking they may be rebuffed. Some take the view that if the doctor wanted them to know he would tell them; some, but few perhaps, do not know that they can ask. Clearly then we must make sure that we allow for this confusion in the relatives' mind and at least inform them of the availability and willingness of the doctor to discuss the illness with them. This can be done by the nursing staff or preferably should be included in information given to the patient on admission. Advice or instruction to patients or relatives may be mistaken or misinterpreted when given verbally, especially at a time of stress, and is best given in a small booklet. The doctor and nurse have difficulties in seeing all patient's relatives and particularly in finding out which is the relative who should be told. Invariably we will have enquiries from the whole family and it is possible that they may not all be told the same thing. We sometimes forget the problems of passing on information; the essential meaning can be altered by changes in intonation, expression, gestures, or by slight variations in phraseology. Added to this we have to consider the reception of information by a worried relative, grasping for hope, suspicious, unfamiliar with many of the words used, and who may have a limited ability to understand even simple language. The doctor has a responsibility to make sure that such relatives do understand. The husband or wife is usually told, but not always; ill health, old age, mental instability, nervousness, inability to cope with the information, etc., may all be factors which need to be considered. The parents will obviously be told when a child has a malignant disease. A big problem arises with the patient who has no relatives and who obviously needs someone to care. Telling relatives calls for discussion and co-operation between several people, the family doctor who is familiar with home circumstances, the consultant, and a medical social worker.

The reactions of the relatives to the information may be more marked than those of the patient; again we are dealing with fear and ignorance together with frustration, anger, resentment, sympathy, and so on. Behind these there is only too often an accusation or objurgation, sometimes of the doctor, but this can be resolved when the facts are discussed and indeed may never have arisen if this had been done earlier on.

Visiting hours in hospital do require the co-operation of the relatives who should be advised to discuss this with the nursing staff. A bed may be surrounded by a variety of friends and relatives of all ages, all rapidly talking and seeking the patient's full attention, albeit with the best intention of keeping him amused and cheering him. But good intentions are not enough. Florence Nightingale has a chapter in *The Art of Nursing* (1859, new edn 1946) entitled 'The Vicious Visitor', in which she says, 'I would appeal most seriously to all friends, visitors and attendants of the sick to leave off the practice of attempting to "cheer" the sick by making light of danger and exaggerating probabilities of recovery. The fact is that the patient is not "cheered" at all by these well-meaning, most tiresome friends.' Written in 1859, there is some excellent advice given in her chapter, which we can consider further. 'How little the real sufferings of illness are known or understood. How little does anyone in good health fancy him or even *herself* into the life of a sick person.' 'A sick person does so enjoy hearing good news.' 'The sick don't want you to be lachrymose and whining, they like you to be fresh and active and interested.' 'There is no better society than babies and sick people together for one another.' 'No mockery in the world is so hollow as advice showered upon the sick – it is possible that the patient has heard such advice at least fifty times before, and that, had it been practicable, it would have been practised long ago.' Bring all this up to date, rephrase it in modern idiom, and you still have good advice.

The Patient at Home

Whilst the patient may prefer to go home at the earliest opportunity, this may not always be convenient to the relatives, who may be elderly, insecure, unable to cope, or incapacitated themselves. Here we have a great problem which if not carefully handled may cause upset to both patient and relative. It also may be undesirable to send the patient home because facilities may be inadequate. Much can be done to help by advice from the family doctor, the district nurse, a social worker, or the social welfare service, together with help from voluntary organizations. Considerable help may be given by other relatives and friends and in some communities by volunteers willing to assist those in need. These various facilities do appear to be somewhat fragmented and not correlated at times. Each service is responsible to different bodies. It sometimes appears that such services are unaware of the need in the community and the patient and his relatives are unaware of the facilities which are available. This could be due to many causes: the desire of patient or relative for independence, the magnitude of the problem for the charitable organizations, or merely a lack of communication. There is an obvious need for a co-ordination of such facilities, but to achieve this we must first determine the patient's needs and also those of the relative at home. In co-ordinating we shall inevitably cut across personal relationships and this is likely to produce embarrassment, with a reluctance to give full information, and will inevitably create a desire to cope without outside help. When these artificial barriers are broken down we shall probably be surprised to find that in many cases worry has been caused unnecessarily and could have been prevented or easily relieved if only the right authorities had known. The community also has a relationship with those who are ill, distressed, or in need. In many cases the best place for the cancer patient is at home, both during his treatment and in convalescence or terminally, the exception being when there is a special need for certain care or treatment which can be obtained only in hospital. The community must accept its role or responsibility and make genuine efforts to help the patient and his relatives. Community hospitals have a definite place for the care of these patients, especially in the terminal stage of the disease, relatives are close at hand, and the family doctor – frequently a friend and known well – is there to take charge. This personal atmosphere is preferable to the somewhat more impersonal approach of the large hospital some distance away, which is necessary only to bring together specialized techniques of treatment or patient care which cannot be disseminated because of expense or because of specific expertise. Organized branches of the community need to examine their role: whether they should give positive help to those in need or are prepared merely to sympathize. If the former, they can then inquire whether a co-operative approach with similar bodies may not be more useful than the somewhat limited help that each can give.

Loneliness can have a detrimental effect; whilst the patient may be at home in his own familiar surroundings the family may be away for long periods of the day, and the consequent boredom leads to introspection. His distress may not be relieved by a mass of people coming home in the evening and asking such questions as 'what have you been doing all day?', over-acting by their fussiness, continuously talking or making a noise as if the excessive attention he now receives will compensate for that which he has not had all day. This is unsatisfactory; equanimity and inexcitability are important, but not silence followed by excessive noise and interference. Radio and television go far to relieve boredom and add variation and, of course, there is always the possibility of turning it off, and on again, as he wishes.

Rehabilitation

The role of the relatives in returning the patient to a normal or near normal life has been inadequately understood in many illnesses but most of all in cancer. Relatives accept the presumed terminal nature of the illness and from then on the patient is shielded from everyday life, is not allowed to do anything for himself, is discouraged from taking part in home life and prevented from doing anything that the relatives think could be done by them or which they consider to be detrimental to his health. Admittedly in most cases this is with the good intent of relieving the patient, but unfortunately it goes further. He feels he is no longer considered as an individual, is ignored in decision-making, no longer has a use, and is 'on the way out'. He is repeatedly made aware of his uselessness, any desire he had to return to normal is thwarted, it becomes easier to give in and accept rather than to struggle back to normal life, especially when his physical condition prevents his full return. All convalescent patients need some incentive, and, indeed, we all need a little 'bullying back to normal' when we have been ill. The wise wife or mother knows that she has much to offer in this way and she bullies with the patient's best interests in mind. Not so with the cancer patient; we get such remarks as 'Incentive? What for? He is dying, let us make him comfortable', and 'Let us organize our work, the family, and the house as if he is not here, as it will be soon enough'. The result is a vegetable existence for the patient, of books, papers, radio, television, leading to anorexia, lassitude, listlessness, boredom, insomnia, constipation, muscular weakness, withdrawal – a rapidly decreasing spiral of good health.

Our intention should be to return our cancer patient back to normal; of course, we have different degrees of normality, depending on the nature of the disease, the complications, the sequelae of treatment, the control of the disease, the occupation, etc. But it is possible either

(a) to return the patient to normal life – with little or no residual effect of his disease,

(b) or to return him back to his work which he may be able to manage quite well even though he may not have his previous state of health;

(c) or return him to lighter work;

(d)   or cure his disease, but only at the expense of his being unemployable;

(e)   or control or palliate knowing that he has a limited time before the disease overtakes him.

There are differing approaches to each of these broad groups; thus in those given above,

(a)   we must encourage him to accept that health has been restored and his relatives must be fully aware of this and must co-operate;

(b)   our encouragement is more difficult; whereas in (a) it is a 'once-off' affair, here it must continue every day because failure to persevere at any time may start a downward path of ill health;

(c)   rehabilitation often needs professional assistance from an experienced worker and his trained staff. The family's role is to support and show pleasure that he has achieved so much;

(d)   we are dealing with a difficult group; the patient may lose his pride, he no longer feels useful, he cannot work, he cannot take responsibility for his family, he needs continuous attention and there is a distinct possibility that he may feel useless. As time goes on and tempers become frayed, the spouse who has had to take over the whole responsibility of the household begins to ignore the 'passenger'. Considerable help for the patient is needed often for a long time and the family themselves will need considerable encouragement to carry on;

(e)   if the expectation of life is short it should be made as interesting as possible, shielding will only promote a feeling of uselessness: in any case what are we shielding him from? – from death? New methods of pain control can be instrumental in making him relatively active, often almost to the end; he should be encouraged to enjoy what life he has left to the full – the problem frequently is not that of convincing the patient but of convincing his relatives and friends.

Thus, the relatives have a big part to play, and frequently they are not informed of what they can do and how much they can help; we must forgive them for not inquiring because they have been led to believe that this is inevitably a fatal disease.

DIET
Many relatives have little knowledge of invalid diets and the ways of inducing people to eat. Our present civilization accepts two or three 'good' meals a day, the timing dictated by the factory or work, so large quantities of food are needed for us to survive to the next meal. Frequently meals are fried or roasted and whilst this is acceptable and enjoyed by the healthy it is not what the invalid needs. Several factors affect his appetite, often he is 'off-colour', there may be some toxaemia, especially if he is having radiotherapy – and toxic products, produced as a result of the killing of malignant cells, will be circulating in the blood stream – he is not taking active exercise and thus does not need such a large fuel intake, and often the sight of a large 'normal' meal or the smell of cooking 'puts him off'. Relatives delight in seeing him eat heartily and despair if he does not. The thought of the assault of a large fatty meal on an empty unwilling stomach is obviously nauseating. Small frequent meals or snacks, as many as ten to fifteen a day, are required. These may be nothing more than a sandwich, a small portion of meat, fruit, fish, in fact, if there is no medical contraindication, anything the patient wants, but in small quantity and daintily served. Such meals may be taken at any time and relatives must not be surprised by requests to eat at odd hours; regrettably they tend to remonstrate rather than provide.

Food should be presented as attractively as possible on a plate, and not just heaped up. It is better to give portions which are too small rather than large ones, if he wants more it can be given. Sandwiches and bread should be cut thinly, the crusts removed, and cut into small fingers. Seasoning and condiments should be left to the patient, because although the relatives know his choices, these often change in illness. Food and drinks often appear more tempting when served with thin, pretty, china plates and cups rather than heavy pottery or plastic. A cracked or chipped utensil can often promote a refusal. Quietness is essential at mealtimes; a patient may be dissuaded from eating if there is a loud radio, continued conversations, especially questions, cajoling, or even interruptions by other people just walking about. Substances with a bitter taste often stimulate the appetite, for example, grapefruit juice, burgundy, stout, sherry, and so on, given in small quantities before meals.

Who informs a generation of relatives who have not been brought up with the niceties of diet? We have forgotten the writings of Mrs Beeton and Florence Nightingale on invalid diets. Advice can be given in the out-patient clinic but it takes time and limits the number of patients that can be seen. Relatives may not seek such advice because they presume that they are supposed to know; perhaps we should help by giving written information and providing diet sheets.

DISTRACTIONS

It is not out of place to mention briefly other things that might help recuperation by giving a little stimulus to the patient's mental condition. These can all be arranged by the patient's relatives. Hobbies were once a great stimulus to interest; differing from everyday work, they promoted relaxation, but, unfortunately for many people, they have been replaced by more passive methods: the radio and television. Hospital occupational therapy may offer simple instruction and may open up new vistas for the convalescent patient. Alternatively, friends or relatives can initiate such new ideas and create an absorbing pastime. Occasional outings in a car are very helpful and we forget sometimes that elderly, lonely people do not have this facility. Here are excellent opportunities for relatives to help. Short holidays from home, at convalescent or holiday homes for the disabled, help to produce relationships with others in similar conditions and make the patient realize that there are others as bad or even worse than themselves, thus reducing their self-pity. They also serve as a stimulus to persevere, and, very important, as a rest for the relations. For ladies we have such simple things as hairdressing, a visit to a clothes shop, the use of perfumes and cosmetics, all signs of normal behaviour and stimulants to getting back to health and strength which can be participated in by relatives.

The care of the patient with malignant disease does not end with the definitive treatment. Aftercare is very important; few of us are fully aware of its implications and the needs of both patient and relatives. At present insufficient is being done to help the relatives to understand the needs of the patient and of their essential role in his care and comfort.

Terminal Care

In most cases terminal care of a patient can be carried out at home if adequate facilities are available but about one quarter of patients need special nursing care in the terminal illness. Of course, we must consider the sex of the patient; if the man is ill care is more readily forthcoming from female members of the family than if it is the woman, nursing being a natural instinct of woman. Acceptance of the need to nurse an elderly spouse is normal and failure to do so is unusual. Over the years there has been a steady change in relatives' attitudes. What was once accepted as a responsibility, duty, or even privilege, is now becoming considered a State obligation. Increasingly we are confronted with a relative who requests, even demands, admission of the patient to hospital on varying grounds from "I have work to do", or "I cannot cope", or "I am not well myself", or "I have had a nervous breakdown", to even "It is your responsibility". Now we must admit that there are problems in taking over this responsibility, and that though many would wish to do so, circumstances associated with modern society prevent it. More women are working to supplement the family income, they obviously have to think about the situation after the husband's death, of where the family's finances will come from; they are, therefore, very anxious not to lose their present job. Attitudes to family responsibility do vary over the country; small rural communities show a much stronger 'togetherness' and responsibility than do the more impersonal city dwellers. Much work needs to be done to discover the problems associated with the care of the sick and dying at home and to develop ways of helping and – very important – making known to the general public what facilities are available.

Bereavement

The worries of bereavement often start much earlier than we recognize. A husband patient who is merely questioning unusual symptoms may pass on his anxiety to his spouse, who may begin a chain of thoughts embellished by such considerations as the age of the patient, a knowledge of similar symptoms occurring in other people and the subsequent outcome, a known family history, thoughts of hospitalization, operation, treatment, suffering, lingering death, then a fear of being left alone – she thus progressively imagines the worst and the fatal outcome. Such imaginary excursions are balanced by hard facts and a more optimistic approach, but as there is deterioration and confirmation of one or more aspects, she experiences the whole picture more acutely – this is the state of pre-bereavement.

What was imagination appears to become based on more solid fact and long before he reaches the terminal stage she has experienced bereavement. Thus, eventually she assumes what she considers is her role. This state of pre-bereavement can account for many of the attitudes which may at first appear confusing – disbelief, pessimism, withdrawn approach, and acceptance of the inevitable.

We have a lead to our study of bereavement from *Mourning and Melancholia* by Sigmund Freud (1856–1939); whilst accepting that it was a departure from the normal attitude to life he still considered it to be a natural response, in no way pathological and not requiring medical treatment. His five characteristics of mourning were (a) painful dejection, (b) loss of interest in the outside world, (c) a failure to adopt a new object of love in the early stages, (d) a rejection of any activities not associated or connected with the dead one, and (e) no disturbance of self-respect as occurs with melancholia. He went on further to consider that normal grief is self-limiting, 'time heals', the reality of the happenings around the bereaved all help, and he advised against any interference, which could disrupt normal recovery and indeed may be harmful.

There are several useful communications concerning the emotions of the bereaved and measures that can be taken to help them over a very difficult period, and J. Hinton has successfully summed these up in his book *Dying* (1972). Grief is, of course, a personal response or experience and people react in different ways; to many it is the end and grief may be protracted for many years with no visible recovery. This response is typical of the Victorians, following the example set by their queen, and is still apparent today although by no means as common as it was once. Death is accepted as inevitable, in fact frequently as a relief or release from suffering in the case of cancer patients. We must, of course, distinguish memory from grief; it is possible to retain an active memory and not to be blighted by grief. Stress after bereavement is natural and is reflected in a wish for death by the spouse in the first twelve months after bereavement; this may in part be due to the immediate bereavement but also to the strain inherent during the terminal illness and even back to the time of pre-bereavement. Readjustment after bereavement can be achieved in so many ways that it is impossible to be dogmatic: so much depends on the individual concerned. Some require a certain amount of solitude and shun proffered help with the result that the would-be helper is offended and embarrassed and fails to give help at a time when it really is needed. Some rely heavily on friends or relatives, require constant attention and company, and in some the reaction is almost psychotic and may need medical attention. What is required is a sympathetic approach by all who come into contact with the bereaved person. Sympathy can be shown in many ways, for example, by being quiet when this is needed, by making a cup of tea, or merely by a friendly handshake, for these can frequently be of more help than a verbal 'post mortem' on the case or a raking up of memories. Everyday affairs must be looked after and the adoption of a normal routine will often help to allay the grief. Relatives can help by keeping up an interest in the normal, remembering holidays, family occasions, birthdays, anniversaries, and so on. Those wishing to help the bereaved must not be embarrassed or put off if they make a mistake or say the wrong thing. Deliberate avoidance of the deceased's name can often produce an artificial situation which further adds to the distress. As far as possible the helper should try to act as normally as he can.

The family doctor or nurse may help by giving a quiet factual account of cancer: what it is, what are the possible causes, why we don't cure every case, the impossibility of life proceeding with certain types of cancer, and the like. Even in times of stress some people find comfort when presented with true facts, especially if they are encouraged to discuss those problems which have confused them, such as techniques of treatment. Let us take as an example a patient who had a cancer of the lung which had spread to his brain and was causing cerebral symptoms; we may be asked why was the brain also given radiation treatment when the trouble was in the chest. Such treatment was accepted at the time when there was a possibility that anything the doctor did could save the patient's life, but after his death inquiry produced questions – did he die because the brain was treated? – surely this was wrong when his complaint was in the chest? – did the doctor do wrong? Involved as the doctor is with treatment and in the full knowledge of the disease, his actions seem quite logical to him but not to the relative, for whom a little time spent in explanation may do much to help.

MEMORY

Some aspects of memory are not fully appreciated; the dead do not grow old in the memory of the bereaved. I know of no better way of expressing this than that given by Charles Dickens (1812–70), in *The Old Curiosity Shop*, written in 1840:

> She was looking at a humble stone which told of a young man who had died at twenty-three years old, fifty-five years ago, when she heard a faltering step approaching, and looking round saw a feeble woman bent with the weight of years, who tottered to the foot of that same grave and asked her to read the writing on the stone. The old woman thanked her when she had done, saying that she had had the words by heart for many a long, long year, but could not see them now.
> 'Were you his mother?' said the child.
> 'I was his wife, my dear.'
> She the wife of a young man of three-and-twenty!
> Ah, true! It was fifty-five years ago.
> 'You wonder to hear me say that,' remarked the old woman, shaking her head. 'You're not the first. Older folk than you have wondered at the same thing before now. Yes, I was his wife. Death doesn't change us more than life, my dear.'
> 'Do you come here often?' asked the child.
> 'I sit here very often in the summer-time,' she answered.
> 'I used to come here once to cry and mourn, but that was a weary while ago, bless God!'
> 'I pluck the daisies as they grow, and take them home,' said the old woman after a short silence. 'I like no flowers so well as these, and haven't for five-and-fifty years. It's a long time and I'm getting very old!'
> Then growing garrulous upon a theme which was new to one listener though it were but a child, she told her how she had wept and moaned and prayed to die herself, when this happened; and how when she first came to that place, a young

creature strong in love and grief, she had hoped that her heart was breaking as it seemed to be. But that time passed by, and although she continued to be sad when she came there, still she could bear to come, and so went on until it was pain no longer, but a solemn pleasure, and a duty she had learned to like. And now that five-and-fifty years were gone, she spoke of the dead man as if he had been her son or grandson, with a kind of pity for his youth, growing out of her own old age, and an exalting of his strength and manly beauty as compared with her own weakness and decay; and yet she spoke about him as her husband too, and thinking of herself in connexion with him, as she used to be and not as she was now, talked of their meeting in another world, as if he were dead but yesterday, and she, separated from her former self, were thinking of the happiness of that comely girl who seemed to have died with him.

We are fortunate that as time passes we remember the happier times rather than the sad. Terminal illness may frequently be distressing to those remaining; associate this with a realization that the illness is cancer and this distress is increased. In the early days of bereavement distress is a very painful memory, but as time goes on it becomes less important and may be forgotten. In time the remaining memory is not of a dying relative but of a living, active, vital one. Small wonder then that poets use such adjectives as 'fond', 'dear', 'sweet', 'fair', and 'bright' when talking of memory.

The wise friend will try to assist this memory be recalling past events which gave pleasure or by producing photographs; of course, such action must be at the appropriate time and with the relative's co-operation.

At one time memory appeared to be centred on a material thing – a grave, a tombstone, and the prevalent practice of the weekly floral tribute. Present-day society has changed its ideas, perhaps as a result of the increased use of cremation, of excellent photographs, of a decreasing desire for the materialistic, or merely as a result of changing ideas.

The Young Relative

We have a better approach to our children now than was evident even thirty or forty years ago. The policy that children should be seen and not heard, adopted because it avoided the embarrassment of explanation, has fortunately been replaced with one of discussion and involvement of the child.

The trauma of death to a child can be unimaginable; to see a parent who was lively, authoritative, always present, begin to show signs of failure and ill-health obviously brings some realization of the severity of the disease to the child. To find that the parent is no longer there brings despair and then to have questions unanswered or incompletely answered adds even further to the child's problems. 'Gone away' raises hopes of return. 'Gone to live with Jesus' brings the response 'Why? I need her more than him'. 'Gone to Heaven' creates a feeling of unreality, disbelief, the unknown. We sometimes forget that the child cannot imagine abstract things in the same way that the adult can; his fantasy is associated with the happenings of reality – fairy tales are often based on fact or at least on situations associated with fact and they involve material things and persons – fairies, giants, maybe, but material and imaginable based on human form. Heaven is vague – where is it? – who has seen it? – The problems of the child who loses his parent are neatly summed up in a poet's description of his own traumatic experiences:

> Thy maidens, grieved themselves at my concern,
> Oft gave me promise of thy quick return,
> What ardently I wished, I long believed,
> And disappointed still, was still deceived,
> By expectation every day beguiled,
> Dupe of tomorrow even from a child,
> Thus many a sad tomorrow came and went,
> Till, all my stock of infant sorrow spent
> I learned at last submission to my lot
> But, though I less deplored thee, ne'er forgot.

(William Cowper (1737–1800), *On the receipt of his mother's picture*)

Although the child may show a quick reassertion of his normal life to his friends, he may suffer an unconscious loss and develop a resentment that his parent left him when he was unprepared. William Cowper's mother did in fact die when he was six years old and this had a lasting effect on him, which in part may account for his behaviour in later life: one of trouble, sorrow, and mental disturbance. His poem also brings out the need for a material remembrance – a likeness – a picture of the deceased. Adults with accumulated years of visual memory of the bereaved often forget that the child has no such store and fails to evoke a mental image. Here then is the importance of keeping family photographs.

In cancer we have a disease running a somewhat chronic course so that there is usually time to prepare the child and for the child to see the effect of the disease on the parent. The realization of the nature of the disease with some idea of its inevitable progress will prepare him and he will inevitably respond by giving the attention and thought that a parent needs at this time. Many children can give considerable help in the home, can comfort the spouse, be quiet when requested to, and join in discussion and action when needed. Perhaps unconsciously the child will also appreciate that the parent is ill, even suffering, and that death is a 'happy release' from suffering.

The Childrens' Responsibilities

It is often assumed that the old, ill person is delighted at the prospects of living with a son or daughter, but this is not always so. Frequently they wish to keep some independence and should be encouraged to do so as long as possible. This can be arranged if the family lives near and can call in daily. However, there comes a time when this is no longer possible and the children need to have some plan worked out with the patient's own doctor for the future. This will require the full use of the social services and possible admission to a nursing home, local hospital, or terminal home.

It is important to recognize that, today, living with one's children is often an unnatural condition brought about by old age, incapacity, illness, and dependence. Such conditions frequently promote distress or at least stress, and there need to be safety valves for such a situation. In many cases there is happiness and serenity and this is more likely to be achieved if the relatives can have a certain degree of independence; but this may not be possible and the patient has to be integrated into a busy home. Inadequate facilities or overcrowding produce volatile atmospheres and stress, or even suffering. Breaks are needed for both the patient and children and it would be desirable if the patient could be taken into a home for a short rest from time to time. This could take the form of a holiday home rather than an institution or geriatric ward which frequently is the only accommodation that we have to offer.

Offensive discharges or wounds and growing visible tumours are distressing and embarrassing. Toilet facilities, bed-pans, and incontinence produce special problems or embarrassing situations. All are exaggerated when inquisitive or sensitive young grandchildren are present in the house. People who were grumblers and awkward when young are frequently so in old age; they can make life unbearable, criticizing children, having the radio or television turned on full because they are deaf, but refusing at the same time to wear an effective deaf-aid, and so on, until even the most loving of families can reach breaking-point.

It is frequently presumed that an unmarried member of the family, especially a daughter, will want, or even have a duty, to nurse those who are older or sick. But even single people have ties and responsibilities and often are building up their own lives. Unmarried daughters can and should be helped by other members of the family. These should take their turn in nursing, or take the parent into their homes if possible, or move into the family home to give their sister an occasional holiday. For the unmarried daughter to be responsible for the whole burden is unfair, to lose her chance of future marriage or happiness is unthinkable, and yet it occurs. Any attempt to resist that responsibility inevitably fills her with remorse.

The *only* child faces even more problems with fewer alternatives; without doubt such people need help, as their plight often goes unrecognized or ignored. In an age when security and welfare have become the responsibilities of the state or community the needs of the children must also be considered. It is inevitable that when taking on responsibility for a cancer parent the child often thinks that this will be for a short time only. Recovery or partial recovery of the patient does not always leave him in a condition capable of being rehabilitated to normal life; or he may be afraid, unprepared, and quite happy to go on in his new guise of dependence. The child too is uncertain that the parent is cured, imagines recovery to be impossible, and goes on from one week to another, one month, one year, without limit, always afraid to resume her independence in case death is just around the corner, unwilling to shirk responsibility – after all, is it not cancer? Public education, willing helpers, social services, will go far to correct these attitudes.

Wherever the cancer patient is spending his last days there is, unfortunately, a feeling of caring or paying attention to a terminal disease. It is regrettable that the term 'terminal care' has been coined; it no longer implies care of a person, but disease care, and suggests that there is some uniformity about the end result of malignant disease. We need to concentrate more on the patient rather than on the disease state – not a terminal case of cancer of the breast, lung and so on, but my mother, or my father. Thus, even in the family home the children may need to be reminded of their relationship to the patient, and over-familiarity or off-handedness comes badly at this time. Perhaps the very nature of the illness makes children reject the person. 'This cannot be my mother – it is someone sick and dying of cancer.' Perhaps this is an unconscious way of reducing involvement, or possibly it relieves the strain of seeing one's own parents die or suffer. Perhaps it is because at this time the parent appears to lose the dignity which the child has always associated with him. At times the child will need to be reassured that the parent's cancer is not 'catching' and that there is no evidence that this is a hereditary disease.

The daughter may have a further problem of communication with her parent because illness sometimes raises artificial barriers between relatives. She may have been told the true nature of the disease but is unable to discuss this with her parent. The parent too may suffer to see the child worried; at times he knows the diagnosis but is afraid to discuss it with the child because of worrying her.

Death is an essential part of life, albeit inevitable and final. The relatives' reaction will depend on so many factors, the age of the patient, the relationship, any suffering experienced, and the like. The preparations they have made will also depend on many factors, such as personal beliefs, their religion, or attitudes which suggest that the dead are better off and may be enjoying a better life. Christian beliefs can, or at least should, prepare for this, and in many cases do.

Much of what we have said about relatives applies also to close friends and acquaintances who are not such disinterested observers as are the general public.

12
Current Attitudes of the Public

It is a common human failing that we are unable to appreciate the misfortunes of others when our thoughts are so full of our own; Joseph Addison (1672–1719), in *The Mountain of Miseries*, describes his dream inspired by reading Socrates. Fancy, a lady of thin airy shape, by order of Jupiter, takes the burdens of misfortune from each man's shoulders and collects them on a plain. Jupiter then decrees that every man will exchange his affliction and take up another. So, 'the poor hunchback went off a very well-shaped person with a stone in his bladder', a poor galley slave threw off his chains and took up the gout, and so on. But these exchanges only produced further complaints and lamentations until Jupiter, taking pity, sent Patience to return to every man his own calamity with which he was contented. And so:

> I learnt from it never to repine at my own misfortunes, or to envy the happiness of another, since it is impossible for any man to form a right judgement of his neighbour's suffering; for which reason also I have determined never to think lightly of another's complaints, but to regard the sorrows of my fellow creatures with sentiments of humanity and compassion.

We are all guilty of thinking we have all the worries and that others are better off. But not so with cancer; it surely is a measure of the hopelessness or gravity of the disease in the public mind that no one considers the cancer patient to be better off or that he himself is worse off than the cancer patient. None would change places. Cancer thus holds a place of respect; all people pity the patient with it, and pity also the family of that man.

We may now examine how members of the general public react when they hear that someone has cancer. In the first place there is relief – 'It may have been me!', or 'Thank God I haven't got it!' This is followed by a feeling of sympathy which is no more than a natural response of all normal people towards others in distress. But sympathy may be in the mind only, it may evoke a verbal response, a few kind words; only occasionally does it become practical and give help. Alas! More often than not it incites only the response of sending flowers to the funeral or a donation to charity in lieu.

The news evokes also a mixture of curiosity and expectation; here is a man with cancer, therefore he will obviously go downhill and eventually die and we can exclaim 'I told you so', because, of course, we know what is inevitable. If the expected does not happen it is 'obvious that it was not a cancer', because 'those people that I have known with cancer have all died'. Now, possibly this is true for that individual observer because the word *cancer* is seldom or never mentioned in those patients who survive. But, because of lack of knowledge, he is not justified in concluding that '*all* patients with cancer die from their disease'. And this is the conclusion that the general public often reaches, out of ignorance of the true facts. Mrs Smith goes into hospital, has an operation or treatment and comes home, goes steadily downhill and dies – 'It was *cancer* you know'; whereas a neighbour with the same disease, at the same stage, goes into hospital, has the same treatment, is ill for a time then improves, and the word *cancer* is never mentioned.

Small wonder then that everything is loaded against the disease; it is only mentioned when death occurs, but why not in the cured case? Frequently the patient does not know, the relatives, even if they do know, may not want to mention it, either because it may upset the patient or because they imagine that the disease has some form of social stigma.

The general public appear to have an unusual attachment to the very word *cancer*; this word means something, whereas synonymous words do not have the same meaning. Thus, there is often no fear when such terms as 'tumour', 'carcinoma', 'malignancy', or even 'growth' are used, and these words do not appear to have the same association with death. Frequently we see relief, albeit misplaced, when in attempting to break the news to relatives we use a synonymous term – 'Oh, thank goodness it is not cancer'. Some people will accept the word radiotherapy without connecting it with cancer; perhaps the term *therapy* implies an innocuous association as a result of its use in physio*therapy*, hydro*therapy*, and occupational *therapy*, all of which deal more usually with non-malignant diseases and are known to produce cures.

Suffering, pain, offensive discharges, distress, are thought to be invariable accompaniments to this disease and many people can give a vivid description of such suffering. This is in contradiction to the findings of many doctors, either in general practice or in hospital. If there is no suffering we may find that the word cancer is not mentioned.

The general public is only familiar with the established disease, at present only little progress has been made in educating them in its detection, appreciation of suspicious symptoms, and the realization of aetiological factors which could lead to its prevention. Witness the poor results of campaigns aimed at abolishing smoking. Disbelief, knowledge of someone – usually Winston Churchill – who has smoked 'like a chimney all his life', a belief that it is 'something that happens to someone else, not me', and the teenager's view of 'what does it matter, twenty, thirty, or forty years on is a lifetime', is not going to worry them. These are all attitudes of non-acceptance of the facts which indicate that it is wrong or harmful to carry on a practice which is giving pleasure. Thus we get involved with individualistic attitudes or rights of the individual; even more, a rugged determination to 'do it if I want to', and 'who are you to interfere or advise me?'

If we ask members of the public what they know of cancer we will find many varied responses; the young are uninterested, the middle-aged too busy, but the elderly have different ideas – they know friends and acquaintances and fear it may come to them. Again we may find differences due to sex, to educational standards, to social status, to geographical factors, to current views, reports, and much else. Many surveys have been made of the general public's opinion, but we must be cautious in interpreting them because they represent only the findings in a selected group of people, at a certain place, at a precise period of time, and we must resist any temptation to draw conclusions or to generalize.

The public attitude is complex and affected by many factors. Much is based on surmise and hearsay, and there is an obvious need for the presentation of facts in ways that can be appreciated easily with little or no background knowledge.

13
Possible Solutions

It is, of course, much easier to detail problems than to suggest remedies. Cancer produces these problems because we have no definite panacea – we cannot cure every patient. We have three possible ways of dealing with these problems; to improve the cure rate so that the disease no longer holds the dread it now does, to promote a better understanding of the care that already exists, and to help the sufferer and his family.

Cure

Medical history abounds with details of calamities, epidemics, pandemics, and scourges which once struck dread into every man's mind. Even today, when we read of thousands dying from plague, smallpox, malaria, or cholera, we can appreciate the fear that the possibility of infection by these diseases produced. There was no known cure, and our forefathers resorted to unorthodox treatments or made desperate attempts to allay the disease's progress: by fervent prayer and atonement, sacrifice to the deities, by magic or witchcraft, and so on – anything to appease or placate. These diseases have been controlled and virtually wiped out by relatively simple public health measures; the control of a disease is possible even though we may not understand it fully or know the causative agent. Older members of the community can still appreciate the fear that surrounded a diagnosis of tuberculosis, pneumonia, appendicitis, and diabetes; now that fear has been removed to a large extent. Some diseases, such as infections, can be completely cured with no residual sequelae; others, such as diabetes, are controlled to such an extent that the patient can have normal life expectation. It is reasonable to suggest that if we cure all cases of cancer, that too would no longer be considered a scourge. Regrettably there are few cancers in which we can claim a complete cure; we have a range of survival rates depending on the type of lesion, the site, the clinical staging, the histological pattern, and other factors. We have no reason to be complacent with our results, but over the past few years we are seeing improvements as a result of continuing research.

RESEARCH

We all look forward to the day when cancer can be controlled. As yet we are not sure how that will be brought about and consequently research is undertaken on many fronts. We may be able to establish the cause or causes of cancer and removing these could be the answer; regrettably we have abundant evidence that the general public do not accept advice of this kind. Alternatively we may seek to determine what individuals are more susceptible to carcinogens; we could attempt to get detection of disease or look to ways of improving the treatment of the established disease. Every doctor in his work practises research, the search for knowledge which indicates ways of improving his patient care. Some doctors are, of course, more active than others and have a peculiar bent for this work. We are reminded that good research workers are born rather than made. In this field more than any other the research worker needs to co-operate with workers in other disciplines and in particular with scientists. There are many and varied attitudes to research, the problems of cancer research differ only little from those found in other branches of medicine, and so we will not discuss them further here but concern ourselves briefly with the methods of research which could provide a remedy to our attitudes to cancer by improving the methods of controlling the disease. Such research work may be patient-orientated or laboratory-based.

Patients

Much of our knowledge in medicine has grown up by individual experience, which has suggested that one method of treatment is preferable to another. Often a treatment was accepted because of the seniority of a clinician who advocated it, at times without positive indication of its superiority. Thus, over a period of years we have devised a standard method of treatment which is accepted by the vast majority of the medical profession. This is a slow and somewhat doubtful method of progress. For the treatment of cancer we could offer no more than limited surgery until the turn of this century. Now the scope of surgery has been greatly increased, radiotherapy has established a definite place and more recently so has chemotherapy, and within each of these main treatment parameters we have numerous variations. We now have available many differing treatment techniques and almost unlimited combinations and permutations of these. As a result there are conflicting views from those responsible for treatment, each therapist firmly believing the treatment he has developed to be the best. But there must be some which are better than others, producing better survival with minimal damage to normal tissues. We need, therefore, to search for optimal treatment conditions. The slow evaluation of the results of treatment by clinical impression and experience has been supplanted by the scientific clinical trial with its controls and statistical analyses. Clinical trials may be small, carried out in one institution, or may be co-operative on a regional, national, or even an international scale. Essentially such trials compare two existing treatment techniques in two similarly composed groups of patients and determine whether one method of treatment is superior to the other. Progress is slow as a number of patients need to be collected, treated as indicated, and followed up for a period of time, the indices being survival and complications from treatment. The results of such trials are often not dramatic; often, we are looking for only a small percentage improvement, but all the time we are progressing and the results are improving. It is obvious that such trials produce problems of medical ethics, which may effect the attitudes of the doctors concerned. The medical profession has its own code of ethics; in recent years individual doctors have been helped by advice from learned societies, while in most hospitals such trials are reviewed by ethics committees consisting of doctors and laymen but the final responsibility for deciding whether or not such a trial is undertaken rests with the individual clinician. Such trials have already shown their worth and we have proof that some treatment techniques are preferable to others.

Laboratory
Research work in the laboratory may be associated with the patient, involving blood, serum, or tissue taken from the patient, or may be basic, looking at fundamental concepts which could be applied to the clinical field. In recent years there has been considerable work on the immunological aspects of patients with malignant disease and their response to treatment. This work has progressed to such a stage that we can forecast

that in the not too distant future we may determine that a patient has a cancer before he has symptoms, may even suggest the possible site and type of growth, predict what the response to treatment would be and also determine if and when recurrence occurs. Immunological responses may be used also to develop a resistance in the body to cancer and stimulate the host cells to extirpate the growing malignancy. Biopsy material taken from the cancer can be grown away from the body – tissue culture – and various treatment modes tried out on the cells to aid the clinician in his choice of treatment.

Much laboratory research may appear at first sight to be unconnected with the patient: for example, work involving animals, chemicals in test tubes, material under the microscope, but this basic research helps us to understand more about the normal cell, the body tissues, the cancer cell, and the host response. Such basic research may be referred to as 'curiosity based' or 'fundamental'.

Other research may be involved with aetiological and epidemiological studies to determine the possible causes of cancer within the community, with the aim of removing or reducing incriminated carcinogens and perhaps of preventing some cancers. Methods of detection and early diagnosis have obviously attracted determined research projects aimed at detecting and treating the disease before dissemination has occurred. Careful statistical analysis applied to all aspects of research have enabled us to determine a degree of probability when presenting any results, and such statistical methods have played an important part in research programmes.

Cancer research is developing on a very wide front, progress is being made, and we are learning more each day. We no longer look for a single tablet to cure, such thinking being more applicable to infections caused by one offending organism. Cancer is more complex, and there are many differing forms, each probably needing different therapeutic approaches. Ultimately such research will result in control of the disease, either by prevention or treatment.

Understanding

The two important factors producing our present-day attitudes are fear and ignorance. Both are intimately connected and interrelated; ignorance of the true facts produces and sustains our fears, making them difficult to be removed, fear forces us to deny experience and to accept more basic beliefs. Thus attempts to remove one may be difficult because of the influence of the other. But one can be changed: *ignorance* can be corrected, and this would be the obvious place to start if we are to alter current attitudes.

The word 'ignorance' implies a lack of knowledge which occasionally may be an act of commission – that is, a deliberate attempt to avoid instruction or, more usually, an act of omission in teaching, a state allied to innocence. The first implies some blame to the individual, in the second blame is more correctly apportioned to the community who are ultimately responsible. Where knowedge is lacking we frequently assume that there exists an empty void which is available to be filled. This may be correct in the child and it is just at this age, the formative years, that we attempt to instil basic knowledge. In the adult, however, there is no such void, the mind is already filled with incorrect beliefs or opinions and these have to be removed before new facts are accepted. These beliefs may be no more than simple mis-statements obtained from various sources: 'Cancer is never cured' or 'There is nothing to be done because he has cancer' – information which has been there for many years, accepted mainly because the longer it exists uncorrected the more likely it is to be correct. The intelligence of the individual is not always related to incorrect beliefs, especially if there has been no attempt at determining the true facts or no opportunity to correct false facts. Thus we may find these beliefs in doctors as we do in the general public if the doctor's training has not included these aspects of malignant disease. We must make sure therefore that the doctor has factual information available on which he can base his attitude to cancer, and this information must be available during his formative years of training in the medical school, must continue throughout his post-graduate years, and must become the major part of the training of the specialist interested in malignant diseases. The whole field of medicine is, however, getting wider and it becomes increasingly difficult to keep up to date with all aspects of the subject.

The specialist will need to have a knowledge in depth of malignancies and may even concentrate his interest to one parti- cular malignancy, but there is a danger that he may not be aware of advances being made in allied subjects which could have a bearing on his work. The established specialist relies on the ever-growing mountain of literature to keep him abreast of work, he is helped by review articles, abstracts and indexes of articles, together with some system of library research, but he must be provided with time. The general practitioner needs adequate knowledge of the whole field of medicine, not only of the common diseases, but also of the rarer ones which he may meet. His time for reading is severely limited and he needs well-written, short, informative articles on aspects of malignant disease. He requires details of the frequency of occurrence, possible age groups, symptomatology, diagnosis, and an indication of the best methods of treatment. In recent years we have seen more of these publications aimed specifically at general practitioners.

All doctors need some updating of their knowledge. Those responsible for teaching have the added advantage that they too are taught by their junior staff, or at least brought up to date. Family doctors have appreciated these problems and have taken adequate steps to keep up-to-date at post-graduate centres and by special meetings designed for them.

We sometimes forget how basic is the information required; if there has been little or no undergraduate training in the management of malignant disease we must start at the bottom. Greater co-operation between consultants has resulted in an increased number of combined clinics and the advantages of such clinics are great; they produce a better understanding of patient management and will improve patient care.

We can now turn our attention to the lay public and, as with the doctors, there is a need to educate. We want the general public to have a better appreciation of all aspects of malignancy: the prevention, methods of diagnosis, definitive treatment; such knowledge will help to remove the fear. We must determine what we want them to know, and, of course, it would be easy to say 'everything'. But this is impossible; the general public have not had the training and experience of the doctor and they would be unable to assess, to balance, or to judge. They need to be told selected items in a way that they can understand. We frequently make the mistake of thinking that a lack of medical training means *no* knowledge. This is not so; many have more than a rudimentary understanding of aspects of medicine and cancer and what is told them must be commensurate with their level of intelligence and/or experience. Thus we must adapt our information to the audience who is to receive it.

There are many points to consider in improving the public's

knowledge, the methods by which they are informed, the advice to be given, and amount or degree of information.

METHODS
Information may be dispensed in a number of ways, including:

Family Doctors
To some people the personal approach is all-important and the family doctor spends considerable time in giving such advice. He was an excellent opportunity for talking to the public, of displaying appropriate posters in his waiting-room, of distributing specialized leaflets containing details of vaginal smears, advice to mastectomy patients, etc. The doctor can help by following his own advice; remember, few are persuaded by the doctor who is smoking.

Cancer Information
In this country there are several Cancer Information Centres established to inform the public about all aspects of cancer. They serve the local community and are fully aware of any local customs, beliefs, habits, or fancies. Such centres distribute posters aimed at prevention, detection of suspicious symptoms, give more factual information in booklet or pamphlet form, arrange and address meetings, often with a film and a trained cancer information officer to answer questions. At such meetings the experienced worker can appreciate the hidden questions of the worried patient, or the patient who has suspicious symptoms, and can persuade him to seek medical attention. The work of such centres supplements the work of the family doctor and does not seek to replace him; indeed, doctors are always available to give advice. The staff of these centres become very proficient at assessing the correct level of approach and standard of information.

Schools
Cancer Information Centres aim their work mainly at the adult, but a few are concerned also with the child at school.

Whilst we may change wrong opinions in the adult's mind we would do better to instil correct information right from the beginning in the mind of the child. Programmes aimed at schools could create a healthy attitude to the disease, by stressing the main symptoms, the methods of diagnosis, the treatment that may be given and, most important, by pointing out that it can be cured. Information about epidemiological factors could reduce the contact from these, and stress that prevention is better than cure. The dangers of smoking can be pointed out even to young children, and such information will almost certainly have a greater effect than in the adult who is already 'hooked'. School programmes can introduce cancer into history lessons, pointing out the scourges that have attacked mankind through the ages, the progress made with treatment and diagnosis associated with medical and scientific developments; in geography lessons, describing the incidence of differing cancers in different parts of the world; in science, describing the application of physics to the diagnosis and treatment of cancer, the discovery and use of X-rays; in philosophy or religious instruction discussing the varying attitudes to cancer; in social sciences, detailing the help that can be given to patients and the responsibilities of the community, and so on. Some teaching at this stage could produce a changed attitude by society to the disease at a later date.

Public Lectures
These have little application today; the heyday of the public lecture, given to the community in its spare time, was reached at the turn of the century.

Publications
Articles in popular magazines have tremendous potential and there have been a desirable number of these in recent years. Such articles have to be factual, correct, unemotive, and written in simple, uncontroversial language. They should be written with medical co-operation, but the doctor alone does not have the correct journalistic approach and this should be left to the professional writer, the doctor making sure of accuracy.

Television and Radio
These are obvious fields for the dissemination of information, as both have a regular, almost captive, audience. They must be used intelligently to get simple facts across; long, tedious, and complicated programmes do no more than confuse. We have something to learn from advertising, short, snappy, factual features, presented unemotionally, getting one message over at a time. Longer programmes are likely to be turned off. It is not easy to strike the correct balance, and obviously different types

of programme are needed for different groups. This could be arranged, the more easily assimilated programmes appearing at 'peak viewing times'. All programmes should aim at stimulating further reading or discussion, and could be supported with appropriate leaflets or digests. As yet, we have made little use of these media.

Telephone Communication
This has been tried in some parts of the country, and recorded advice about signs and symptoms requiring medical attention could be organized on a national scale, like the weather or speaking clock service.

So much for the positive approach to dissemination of information. We must take care that such information is carefully thought out and does not lead the public to worry unnecessarily about cancer. We must also take a positive approach to counteract measures designed to encourage the public to take up habits which cause cancer.

We have evidence that tobacco smoking is harmful and that cancers could be prevented. And yet, there is almost unlimited advertising in magazines, on hoardings, and, to a limited degree, on television. We must admit that these advertisements are cleverly worded, and alter with changing times and circumstances. Thus in recent years the 'maleness' of smoking certain cigarettes has been extolled, as demonstrated by the 'exciting life': fast cars, aeroplanes, expensive surroundings, and sport prowess; alternatively it has been suggested that a degree of sophistication can be achieved: the élite gold look, enjoyment of fine art and antiques; or again, more recently, the relative safety of a certain brand, its low tar content, or the 'cool smoke'. Finally, we have the added attraction of coupons to be collected to provide 'fabulous free gifts'.

In recent years there has been a shift in the audience at which the advertisement is aimed. Smoking has shown some decrease in the higher social classes who now need to be enticed back by persuasive, alluring coloured advertisements in the more expensive sophisticated magazines. The unfortunate thing is that in many minds the respectability of the magazine tends to be transferred to the product advertised. Women have been particularly singled out and many good ladies' journals carry whole-page coloured advertisements – small wonder that we are seeing more tobacco-related cancers in women. It would be impossible to stop such advertisements, which improve the economies of the journals, but perhaps we should learn from advertising techniques and publicize the danger of such habits with similar enthusiasm. We would, of course, meet the problems of financial support; those who care for health and the public do not have the same sales incentive.

Support

There is an obvious need for support for the patient and his relatives and this must include both material and moral support.

There may be a need for facilities in the home, and these can usually be provided by the appropriate authorities if they are informed. This means that those who care or help, such as general practitioners, district nurses, social workers, clergy, must be fully conversant with the available local facilities.

Support for the patient's morale is more difficult; it will come from the same workers, together with relatives and friends. Doctor and nurse give factual information, explain why treatment is needed, why the patient does not get well immediately, encourage when necessary, coax, sympathize, even bully, but should always be ready to listen. But such encouragement essentially comes from one who sincerely believes that there is reason for hope. No amount of such talking will succeed if the doctor disbelieves what he says or is insincere – the patient is alerted to look for falseness; long faces, a serious expression, muttered conversations at the foot of the bed, an uninterested approach, or the impression given that there are more important things to do: all lead him to suspect a hopeless prognosis. It is often difficult for the doctor to give this support, more so the inexperienced lay person who only has a hazy notion of the disease, and that often erroneous. Fortunately there are people in the community who have a natural desire to give support, who do not belong to any one profession, religion, or community; all they have in common is a wish to help their fellow men. We must encourage and help such members if at all possible.

Many relatives feel unable to cope with nursing at home but would be willing to try if only they were given some instruction. This can be arranged by community nurses, general practitioners, health visitors, and nurses sent out from hospital.

There exists a strong relationship between terminal homes and the family home and this improves if the relative knows that advice and reassurance are available when needed. It may be useful to invite relatives to the hospital before the patient's discharge to see dressings applied, tracheal suction performed, appliances changed, and so on.

We sometimes forget the burdens placed on the relative, such as the difficulties of providing facilities, of washing clothes or changing beds, even of shopping, and the sleepless nights because of a restless patient or worry. The public can help in many ways – a few minutes spent in the house looking after the sick person whilst the relative goes out is an example. Whilst many people are very sympathetic, they are sometimes unaware of relatives' problems or of how they can help.

The general public need to know when and how to help. Small communities can organize such care as visiting, shopping, sitting in, preferably on some rota system; it is remarkable how no one visits for long periods and then everyone comes at once. In villages there is often a better helping service than is found in the impersonal loneliness of the large city, where no one knows of the need and no one accepts responsibility for his neighbour. Community organizations, including religious bodies, can give tremendous help, but first they need to be told of the need.

The rehabilitation of the patient after treatment has not received sufficient thought; the term 'cancer' is not consistent with rehabilitation in the majority of minds. Communities and relatives can help here. We need to give more thought to the formation of clubs or societies for patients who have had cancer and have been cured, in the same way as they are founded for other diseases, such as diabetes, ulcerative colitis, and laryngectomy patients. There can be little doubt about the good effect on the patient of seeing someone who has had the same disease and has recovered.

The community has a responsibility to support and help its sick and must be made aware of this responsibility. In fact this is what 'community' means – a sharing – each and all of us have a joint responsibility to help our fellow men.

The methods we can use to change the current attitudes can all be summed up in one word, *education*; this is applicable to all concerned, to the research worker, the doctor, those who care for the patient, the relatives, and the general public.

Epilogue

It is not my intention to burden the reader more by mere reiteration; suffice it to attempt a brief conclusion which may induce him to change his attitudes towards cancer.

Throughout history man has been harassed by various scourges; in time these have been overcome only to be replaced by others, and the present one is cancer. With our imperfect knowledge and inherent fear it is inevitable that we always assume the worst possible prognosis. This fatalistic approach is further stengthened by an aura of secrecy that surrounds the disease and frequently permits its mention only in the terminal stages; cures are enshrouded with a silence perpetrated by the clinician, the family and friends, and often unsuspected by the patient. Announcement of the cure of even a small number of patients is disbelieved by the public, discredited by ancillary workers, and treated with suspicion by many medical colleagues. Recourse to mathematical proof only brings further scepticism.

An increase in the number of deaths due to malignant diseases has demanded that research efforts be directed initially to treatment, to earlier diagnosis, and more recently to prevention, in an attempt to control them. But as yet there have been but few attempts at reducing the fear that most people have, because, in spite of all our work, the death rate is still appalling. Some of our attitudes to cancer are basic to our own make-up, but may be changed by various environmental factors. The most important factors are knowledge and experience, but frequently the knowledge we have is incomplete, even misleading. There is an obvious need for dissemination of facts suitable for the audience receiving them, presented clearly and without the usual heavy emotive element. This information must include the fact that permanent cures can be and are made, but we will encounter scepticism until we can be convincing by producing patients who are cured. This frank approach to the disease may induce us to tell some patients that they have had cancer, and to accept the result of their treatment as the usual and not the exceptional. This will become much easier when we can produce much better results; but remember the results we now produce are considerably better than the zero the general public believe. In time the public will come to accept that cures are an everyday occurrence.

Cancer information techniques will in time induce patients to come earlier for treatment with a greater chance of recovery. Much more important, we need to convince people of the possibility of prevention; we are a long way from this at present as is shown by our failure to reduce tobacco smoking.

Education is a slow process, and we cannot hope to change human attitudes in a short time. We must start with the child so that he can grow to be an enlightened adult who will influence his own child.

We have a long way to go. Medical science and research are already attacking these diseases and the result in many malignant diseases indicates an improvement in overall survival. We cannot afford to waste time because we can no longer justify the appalling loss of life or the suffering these diseases produce. Delay caused by ignorance, fear, or any cause increases the possibility of stress and reduces the chance of cure.

I wish that I could end with simple straightforward advice, a real sting in the tail which would change our attitudes to the disease – a disease I know, which I meet every day, a disease which whilst it depresses me stimulates me further to attempt to cure it. I know that treatment works because daily I see patients who have had the disease and who have successfully overcome it. As the years go by the number of such patients increases, cures are now possible which were unheard of some thirty years ago when I started in this specialized field; the research work that is going on leads me to believe, with confidence, that more such cures will take place in the future, and this scourge, as others in the past, will eventually be wiped out.

I have been provocative and critical of you, the reader, I have blamed you, I think not unfairly, for many of the wrong attitudes to malignant diseases; I can only ask you to help by changing these attitudes, by seeking more factual information and accepting this as any other medical disease which can be and is cured, and in some cases even prevented. The responsibility for bringing about this change is yours.